Shine the

Light

For information: **shinethelight.net**

Cover Design: Paul Prizer

Author Photo: Nora Kelleher

ISBN: 9798450219332

First Edition: August 2021

Shine the Light

One Man and a Stratocaster

on a Mission to Help Others

Recognize and Overcome Their Pain

Seamus Kelleher

www.shinethelight.net

For my beautiful Irish Rose

Mary Pat

and our precious children

James, Rory, Nora and Aidan

The Accident

"Sir, you have been in a bad accident and sustained a serious head injury. You are on a medevac helicopter on the way to the University of Pennsylvania Trauma Center." All I could see were the bright lights mounted on the helmets of the medical team. I was convinced these were the proverbial lights you see on your way to the afterlife. The noise of the rotors was deafening, and the steady shaking of the chopper felt like the Cyclone wooden rollercoaster ride at Coney Island.

I knew I was in trouble and asked the medics if anyone else was hurt. They told me no, but I had taken a bad fall down a flight of stairs at Kildare's bar in Valley Forge, Pennsylvania. I said, "Tell my wife, Mary Pat, I wasn't driving my car." When I asked if I was going to be okay, they said, "We are doing everything we can for you—stay with us, sir, and answer our questions as best you can."

It was June 2, 2007. I had been living on the edge of a cliff for many years and finally slipped off—literally and figuratively. A lethal cocktail of alcohol abuse, cigarettes, a stressful corporate job, the worry of being an older dad to four children under the age of 10, living the life of a musician playing 90-plus shows a year with a successful Celtic rock and roll band, teaching a media course at New York University, and recording my first solo album had finally taken its toll.

I was drinking with friends at Kildare's after a show with my band, Blackthorn. As I left the bar, I turned to say goodnight when I took a misstep. I tumbled down a cement stairway, and judging from the bruises all over my back, fractured ribs and a fractured skull, I hit every step along the way.

My drinking partners that night were Bill and Melissa. Bill was a volunteer firefighter and his girlfriend, Melissa, a dental technician. She immediately noticed the blood pouring from the side of my head and insisted I wasn't moved. Bill had an ambulance and police at the bar within minutes. Kildare's was less than a mile from the headquarters of defense contractor Lockheed Martin. Lockheed had a helipad, making it possible to immediately call in a medevac helicopter to transport me to the Trauma Center in Philadelphia. Within an hour of the fall, I was being operated on. I lost a lot of blood and began getting transfusions, but the biggest problem was bleeding on the brain that the doctors couldn't control.

For the first two days in the intensive care unit, the staff woke me every few hours to make sure my brain was still functioning normally. Wires were hooked up to every part of my body. The staff were honest and told me that it was a waiting game. My job was to answer their litany of questions: "Where are you, what's your name, date of birth, what city are you in?" It became an endless repetition day and night as I listened to the low hum of the large machines in the room and the steady beeps from a wall of monitors, hoping the beeping wouldn't stop.

Thanks to the quick action of Bill and Melissa on that fateful night, the miracle workers at the trauma center and my wife Mary Pat who nursed me back to health, I survived the ordeal. Over the course of the next several months, I made a miraculous recovery. During that period, I had plenty of time to reflect on my life up to that point and what it meant—the good, the bad and the downright ugly.

My brush with death brought my mortality into sharp focus. I had a desire to document my life so my kids might know me better if something did happen to me—I had cheated death but didn't know how much extra time I was given.

I began writing this book in 2008, a year after the accident. It started out as a series of humorous tales that occurred during my music career. After a few chapters, it became clear there was more to my story than a recounting of my adventures and misadventures and my brushes with fame—I've been almost famous at least six times during my career.

A recurring theme was my constant struggle with depression and anxiety and—later in my life—battling alcoholism. Conjuring up those memories was painful in many ways. I felt vulnerable and second guessed the wisdom of putting everything down on the printed page. I was close to tears on many occasions as I relived my experiences entering some dark places, often causing me to step away from the writing process for months at a time. But I also felt a great sense of relief. Writing the book allowed me to shake off the emotional baggage that was dragging me down. I was also reminded of how blessed I have been with a wonderful family, dear friends all over the world, and a music career than has spanned six decades.

The first draft of the book was almost complete in 2009, but something stopped me from getting it done. I couldn't finish the book because, if I was being honest, I had to admit I was an alcoholic. Sadly, despite my near fatal accident, I wasn't ready to say goodbye to my best friend, the drink.

I've been sober now since November 1, 2014. My mental and physical health has, for the most part, been good for several years. I share my story with audiences across America in a motivational talk called "Shine the Light," highlighting the struggles that people with mental health and addiction issues face. I also teach courses on Mental Wellness and Suicide Prevention at Texas A&M College of Medicine. I still perform over 150 shows a year.

I tell my story now so the reader will understand there is always hope, even in the darkest of times. My fervent desire is that people will think and talk about mental wellness and addiction in the same way they discuss their physical health. It's time to "Shine the Light" so we can move away from the darkness and finally let go of the stigma attached to mental illness and addiction.

This is not a tell-all book about my life and my family. There are things I choose to keep private out of respect for the ones I love. We all see life through a different lens. What you see in this book is my story and mine alone.

The Broken Years

When I look back on my secondary school years, I can't recall one good memory. From the first day of class until the day I graduated, I hated every minute of school.

For me, Saint Enda's was a dark walled-in fortress a few miles from Galway City in the west of Ireland. The all-boy school had three hundred boarding students and twenty day pupils, of which I was one. St. Enda's or Colaiste Einne, as it was known in Gaelic, was an all-Irish institution drawing mainly on the Gaelic-speaking areas of Ireland like Donegal, Galway, Clare, Sligo, Kerry and Mayo. English was prohibited from being spoken on school grounds unless it was in an academic or artistic context.

Many families didn't own a car and for the ones that did, the roads were often treacherous—especially in wintertime. It was rare for the boarding students to get a visit from home between September, when the school term started, until the Christmas break in late December. The phone system in Ireland was barely functional, so many boarding students were isolated from their families during the school year.

St. Enda's was an old stone building with multiple block-like sections connected by long corridors. Its high ceilings allowed even the most minute sounds to echo through its halls. In the winter months, it was cold and damp with an antiquated heating system constantly breaking down, adding to an already miserable and dreary environment. To this day, when I think of St. Enda's, I can smell burning oil from the giant furnace room, and the odor of burnt potatoes that filled the air from the large kitchen that prepared the food for the boarders.

The embroidered crest on the dark blue school blazers we wore every day said, "Nec Ardua Terrent," meaning, "No difficulty frightens us" or some absolute bullshit to that effect. It should have read, "Beware of a bunch of sadistic bastards masquerading as priests and teachers." Huge red crosses on a white circular background adorned the roof of each block of the school to protect it from being bombed by lost pilots in World War II when the school was transformed into a medical facility. That always struck me as a paradox, when the biggest threat to the students in St. Enda's came from inside the school.

Our first-year class was broken into two sections with 20 or so students in each. On the first day of class, I, along with the other students, was full of anticipation, looking forward to a new chapter in my life. Within a few hours, my hopes were dashed, when the president, aptly nicknamed "Brutus," dragged ten senior students from their seats during assembly and gave them each 12 belts with a big black leather strap. They were caught smoking cigarettes in the school bathrooms. The strap was specially made for the purpose of corporal punishment with reinforced layers of leather glued together to inflict maximum pain without leaving noticeable marks on the skin. Brutus brought the strap back as far as he could, much like a golfer's back swing, before lunging forward and gaining momentum as he focused intently on the small hands of his young targets. The swoosh of the strap pierced the air before the horrible crack of the strap on the students' palms reverberated through the large hall. The students gasped with each consecutive blow but were careful not to overreact as that could lead to an extra beating. As the punishment continued, Brutus was transformed into a raving lunatic.

Brutus was the seventh son of the seventh son—supposedly someone blessed with magical healing powers. Once or twice a month, long queues of people formed outside his office awaiting his miraculous ability to cure everything from cancer to heart conditions. While he was "healing" people on one side of the school, young boys' dreams were being dashed a hundred yards away. But Brutus was not alone.

Another culprit at St. Enda's was a priest we called "Paddy Mad." We believed his erratic and bizarre moods were altered by the phases of the moon. He was the president of the school for a few years during my time there. On one particularly bad day, he gave my best friend, Tom O' Connor, 40 indiscriminate belts of the leather strap, many of them landing on his neck and back. Like Brutus, Paddy Mad's face got redder with each successive blow and the veins on his neck and face looked like they were about to explode. I was horrified then, and still am today, by violent behavior. I was disturbed and shocked with what Paddy Mad was doing to my friend and said, "Fucking stop!" Instantly, I was dragged down to the president's office where I had to call my mother. Mam, as we called her, was a nurse and had just gone to bed after a twelve-hour night shift. I begged the president to wait until Mam slept for a few hours as I knew she had another twelve-hour shift that night. But he insisted she get out of bed and come up to the school.

Mam was in the president's office within half an hour. When she asked what the problem was, Paddy Mad was at a loss for words. During his incoherent rambling, he said I was getting a warning and needed to behave. Unbelievably, he went on to tell my mother I was a lovely young man and never any trouble. The situation made no sense to my mother. She couldn't understand why he made her come up to the school for nothing. Maybe Paddy Mad realized how difficult it was to explain why he had beaten the crap out of a 15-year-old boy a few hours earlier. Or maybe he discovered Mam was a real smart lady who didn't tolerate fools, regardless of whether they were wearing the intimidating black robes and starched white collar of the priesthood.

By far the most terrifying presence in the school was another priest, Dala, a small wiry, miserable waste of a human being. While Paddy Mad was unpredictable as his moods changed by the minute, there were times when he was actually fun and even bordered on being kind. Not so with Dala. He was pure evil, like some horrible remnant of the SS in Nazi Germany. He was the Latin teacher and his egregious behavior, in and outside the classroom, was disturbing on many levels. From day one, he made it his mission to terrify his young students emotionally and physically. He was a sadistic son of a bitch. If he were in any other line of work, he would be behind bars.

When I share my story, people ask why the students didn't tell their parents what was going on. Part of it was that most parents lived several hours away from the school. Even if the boarding students did make contact with home to tell of the horrors happening behind those six-foot walls at St. Enda's, it's doubtful the parents would have done anything. The clergy were hiding under a veil of infallibility in the Ireland of the late '60s and early '70s. The priests at St. Enda's took full advantage of their elevated and protected status and the geographic and social isolation of their young students, knowing they had nowhere to turn.

The school had several lay teachers who, with few exceptions, turned a blind eye to what was happening. Sadly, the situation was not unique to St. Enda's. It was repeated across Ireland, especially when the schools, some of which also functioned as orphanages, were run by the clergy.

To this day, when I run into some of the students who were at St. Enda's with me, I see sadness and regret in their eyes when the topic of our school days comes up in conversation. They, like me, were robbed of those precious years when we should have been learning and growing in a safe environment, free from the fear of being beaten and berated psychologically by a few psychotic individuals who had absolutely no right to be anywhere near young students.

I'm sure there are many who will tell a different story to mine. If you were a native Gaelic speaker, smart and a decent athlete, your experience at St. Enda's would most likely have been much happier than mine. I fell short in all those areas, as did many of the boarding students. Also, for some of the students from the poorer parts of rural Ireland, St. Enda's, even with its drawbacks, provided regular meals and a place where they could socialize with students speaking their beloved native tongue.

A few years ago, I was asked to speak and perform music for the St. Enda's fourth-year students. As I walked into the school for the first time in forty years, the emotions I felt as a young teenager came at me like a storm of piercing hail. I felt a deep anger at what had happened to me and my fellow students. I wanted to ask Brutus, Paddy Mad and Dala one simple question: "WHY?"

Before meeting with the students, Gerry Hanberry, the teacher at St. Enda's who invited me to speak to his class, took me on a tour of the school. We were in the same class through our elementary and secondary education. He knew how I felt about my schooling. He saw the emotion on my face as we visited those classrooms that held such horrible, dark memories, especially the assembly hall where Brutus had doled out that beating on my first day of school, dashing our hopes and dreams of the future. Gerry and I didn't talk much on our walk through the school. He knew I needed time to myself.

During my talk with the co-ed students, I didn't hold back. They couldn't believe some of the stories I told them about my time in St. Enda's. The students had some great questions, some regarding my schooling and some about my career in music. Their faces lit up when I picked up the guitar and played. I envied the excitement and enthusiasm for life I saw in their young faces. I never had that when I was their age. I told them I was so happy to see what was once such a dark place now transformed into a beacon of education thanks in part to the progressive ideology of my friend Gerry and many others like him. I encouraged the students to take full advantage of their wonderful education so they could become the best they could be.

The Escape

When I was 14, I suffered a bad bout of the flu and was confined to bed for a few weeks. In 1968, not everyone had a television set and, if they did, there was only one per household. It made little difference to me as the "telly" only came on in the evening for a few hours and outside of a few cartoons and the odd Disney movie—most of it was news and current affairs, neither of which interested me. There was no internet, Wi-Fi, smart phones, Nintendo, PlayStation or Xbox. I had little interest in reading, so the days were endlessly long. I rigged up an ingenious mirror on the ceiling so I could see the girls passing my house on their way to school. That was the highlight of my day: the girls going to and from Salerno secondary school, a quarter of a mile from our house. I had a few favorites and just seeing them for a fleeting moment was enough to brighten my otherwise dreary days.

A few days into the flu, I noticed a guitar in a see-through plastic cover leaning against the end of the bed. It belonged to my sister Carol but only had three strings. I had been studying piano for five years, so I was able to pick out a tune on one of the strings. The guitar never appealed to me before I got sick, but now I enjoyed the sound and the sensation of plucking the strings. The guitar didn't leave my hands for the next week. Every waking hour was spent getting a little more adventurous.

As soon as I recovered and was able to get up from my bed and out of the house, I went into town to Raftery's, the bike/music/electronics shop, where I got a set of strings for the guitar. The young shop assistant, Mike McMahon, showed me how to put them on the guitar and tune it up. Over the years, he did the same for hundreds of Galway musicians, starting them on their musical journey.

New strings and a guitar pick in tow and fully recovered from the flu, I practiced an hour a day in my bedroom. Within a month, I was up to two or three hours. After three months, it was six hours, every day. St. Enda's had a music room with several guitars belonging to the boarding students. During lunch break each day, I borrowed one of the guitars and played for 15 minutes. After a while, I discovered an ingenious way to get even more practice time. If I pissed off certain teachers, which wasn't hard to do, I was sent outside the classroom to stand in the corridor for the duration of class. That could be dangerous, since Paddy Mad or Dala might be on the prowl and decide to take a swing at you with the leather strap without asking questions. I was willing to take the risk. My two best options for being kicked out of class were religion and math. Once outside, it was a sprint to the guitar room. I identified a great-sounding acoustic guitar, perfect for practicing at low volume so as not to draw the attention and ire of the mad men. The high ceiling provided a perfect reverb chamber where the notes on each plucked string could float through the air like snowflakes. I was experiencing heaven and hell in the same building on the same day.

Damien Hanley was one of my good friends at St. Enda's. He was also a day pupil and a top-class guitar player. He was classically trained and showed me my first few chords. That's all I needed. I was off to the races. I transferred my years of piano theory to the guitar using Damien's chords as my guide. After the initial few lessons, I didn't play with him for several months, but when we did get together, Damien was shocked. I had done more in a short time than most people did in a year, not because I was a prodigy musician, but because my piano training combined with

18

endless hours of practice paid off. I was obsessed with the guitar and knew even at that early stage it would dominate my world for the rest of my life. I had also found my emotional escape from St Enda's.

Mam and Dad

My mother and father met at a dance during World War II when Dad was in the army reserve and Mam was a nurse at the Mater Hospital in Dublin. They got married after the war and set up house in Galway City. Within six years, my four sisters and I arrived on the scene. We are all just a year apart with me being the youngest.

Dad was one of 12 children raised on the family farm near the town of Dingle in County Kerry. Two of those children died in infancy and Maurice (my middle name) died as a young child.

Dad moved to Galway in his early 20s and worked at the Galway City post office. He had a great head on his shoulders, with the ability to read the daily newspapers each morning and synthesize the information in the most pragmatic way. He could have a well-informed conversation on just about any topic.

Dad was also a natural leader. He was chairman of the Salthill Tourist Association and way ahead of his time in terms of marketing the seaside resort, two miles from Galway. He was also active in the post office union and served as chairman of a committee that was rebuilding Christ the King Church in Salthill.

My mother was one of six children. She was born in Cavan and moved to Dublin in her late teens to study nursing at the Mater Hospital. Mam almost died after I was born in 1954. She suffered from ulcerative colitis, which at the time was a deadly disease. She underwent surgery and, according to my sister Maura, there were prayers being offered all over Galway for her recovery. She was blessed to have the best of care and was the beneficiary of a brand-new antibiotic called tetracycline. The surgeon's wife drove to Limerick, a two-hour trip each way from Galway, to pick up this new wonder medication for Mam. Before the surgery, the doctor told her she had a fight on her hands. Mam said she had everything to live for with five kids under the age of six.

I can only imagine the stress Dad experienced with his beautiful young wife battling a deadly illness and five children to look after, while holding down a busy and high-pressure job at the post office. Thanks to the talented medical team and her determination to fight for her life, Mam's treatment was successful and over the course of a year she fully recovered.

She stayed at home to take care of us when we were young. She was an amazing cook and could make a gourmet meal out of anything. She was known for her Sunday roast dinner. Sadly, I was a terrible finicky eater and never ate one of the wonderful meals she prepared—one of my big regrets in life. I broke her heart and Dad's because of my struggles with food. I survived on eggs, chips (French fries), sausages, beans and toast, and the mouth-watering brown bread Mam made sure was always on hand so I would eat something healthy. Yes, I was spoiled rotten by my mother. What I would give to sit down today to one of her Sunday dinners and savor the aromas of her roast potatoes and the sauces she created out of nothing. My sisters were old enough to learn Mam's culinary skills so through their lovely meals, I get a glimpse of what I missed out on.

Mam was also a skilled seamstress and often made matching outfits for my sisters. My wife, Mary Pat, is also a great seamstress and when I hear the sound of her sewing machine, it brings me back to when my sisters and I watched TV with the intermittent hum of the Singer sewing machine in the background. My favorite spot to sit during the long Irish winters with the gale force winds and rain coming off the wild Atlantic was on the floor in front of the roaring fire propped up by the arm of the sofa next to Mam's sewing machine.

Mam, like Dad, had a great sense of humor and was always the center of attention without ever trying. Our kitchen was the confessional for the neighborhood. Everyone from our next-door neighbors to my piano teacher was invited into the kitchen for a chat and the "cuppa tea."

My sisters' friends congregated around our kitchen table most Saturday mornings, often before my sisters got out of bed, just to chat with Mam and seek her advice on how to deal with their latest romance drama, or just to talk about life. She was a great listener with endless empathy and compassion for people. I don't ever remember her saying a bad word about anyone. She found the positive in every person and in every situation.

Because of her medical training, Mam was often called upon to help the sick and the dying. Back then, people were waked in their homes, and she bathed old folks and laid them out after they died.

In the 1970s, Galway had a large population of what we referred to then as "tinkers" or "gypsies," who lived in makeshift tents on the side of the road. Today, this population is known as the "Traveller" community. They are descended from a nomadic culture dating back hundreds of years.

There were two traveller families living near us in Salthill, the McDonaghs and Wards. Both were large, with well over ten children each. Much like the Hatfields and McCoys in America, they were constantly feuding, and alcohol was a big part of their culture. It was hard to watch the young children living in flimsy tents by the side of the road in squalid conditions, especially during the cold, wet and windy Irish winter. It was not uncommon to get a knock on our door in the middle of the night with several kids outside telling us that their mam and dad had not come home from the pub. My parents, sisters and I always jumped into action to do what we could for the poor children.

Many a day, upon my return from school, I saw Mam bandaging one of the traveller children, who were prone to all kinds of physical ailments and infections because of their miserable living conditions. Those kids never left our doorstep without some hot scones, fresh baked brown bread and biscuits.

Over the years, we took in aunts, uncles, cousins, just about anyone from all over Ireland, England and as far away as America. Sometimes it was someone who came to stay for days and lingered for a year for no particular reason. There were times when our house was a safe place for individuals struggling with the cards they were dealt. Mam and Dad treated each new arrival as one of the family. The ones who struggled were helped back on their feet. With the five of us to take care of and the constant stream of visitors, finances were often strained, but as children we never knew it. Even with a full house, as was often the case, we had everything a child could ask for. At an early age, we learned to share what we had and treat all people with respect and dignity regardless of color, creed or class. We had an obligation to help those less fortunate.

Charming Salthill

Salthill, where we grew up, was a beautiful, charming seaside resort two miles from Galway City. As kids, I don't think we fully appreciated what we had at our doorstep. We lived in a row of twelve semi-detached houses built in 1959. Everyone moved into the development around the same time. Most of the families had young children so there was a great sense of community and plenty of friends our age to play with. There was a football stadium directly across from our front door where my friends and I played ball all day long. We also had orchards and wild wooded areas within a few hundred yards of the house where we played elaborate games.

Our house was six hundred yards from the beach with a beautiful promenade stretching two miles where you could look out over Galway Bay to the lovely hills of Country Clare in the distance. It was simply idyllic, but I never bothered to look across at those spectacular hills and appreciate the wildness or tranquility of the bay. I don't ever remember watching the world-famous beautiful sunsets on Galway Bay. I was a young fella and had other things in mind.

Living in a seaside resort, we had access to great summer job opportunities. Dad was well known in Salthill and liked by everyone, so a word from him got you an interview with potential employers. My first job was at age 13 washing dishes in a hotel. I remember the horrible smell of old food and dirty dishes. The hotel manager often came into the kitchen and inspected the dishes telling me to wash them all again if he found as much as one dirty spot on a dish. Things changed for the better at age 14 when I got a job as a waiter in the Oslo Hotel, a hot spot in the middle of

Salthill during the summer months. The centerpiece of the hotel was a cabaret room accommodating over 300 guests. The head bartender, Christy Higgins, was a legendary figure in the Galway bar scene. He took me under his wing and was very good to me, as were the owners Frank and Michael Hallinon.

The hours were long at the Oslo and the work hard, but it was good for me as I was forced to interact with hundreds of people every night, something that I was not very good at prior to that. The work also allowed me to step away from my newfound obsession with the guitar for extended periods of time.

I heard amazing musicians in the cabaret room each night. After work, I went to the Seapoint Ballroom across the street from the Oslo to hear the showbands that performed nightly. I experienced some of Ireland's best guitarists up close. Most of the time, the doormen at Seapoint let me in for free. Based on what I was wearing and the state of me, they knew I wasn't there for the dancing. I was there to learn my craft from the very best.

Magic in a Bottle

In autumn of 1968, I got a call from my friend Damien Hanley asking me to play music, or "jam" as we called it, at his house. We immediately hit it off and he treated me like a peer rather than his student, as was the case when we played together previously. I played harmonica and guitar and he played guitar and sang. Soon after that, through a friend of Damien, we were hired to do a "Cultural Evening" at a Jesuit secondary school in town. We had to learn five songs. It was easy to choose the music as we both loved Creedence Clearwater Revival and a group from England called the Tremeloes. Damien and I never talked much; we just read each other's minds and picked out our parts. Those were wonderful moments of discovery for us. Despite Damien's classical training, he let me go off on my wild playing. The chemistry between us was powerful. It was "magic in a bottle."

On the night of the gig, I was sorry I agreed to do the show. I couldn't eat all day and I was shaking at the very thought of getting up in front of people—forget about playing music. St. Enda's was an all-boys school and it was rare to see a female form in the vicinity of the school. So, it was a shock when I arrived at the cultural evening to see equal numbers of girls and guys, and that some were even holding hands—grounds for immediate expulsion at St. Enda's.

I looked out from the stage and saw over a hundred people with their eyes focused on Damien and me. My knees were literally weak but after the first few chords of "Proud Mary," I knew we were connecting with our audience as I could see heads shaking and bobbing to each note we played.

Halfway through the performance, the nerves settled down and I was overwhelmed by a feeling of joy I had never experienced before.

The first time you feel yourself connecting with another musician in front of an audience, it's like discovering sex. It's scary, exciting, you're glad—or at least relieved—when it's over, and you can't wait to do it again. The night went well and we got a great reception. I consider the show with Damien that evening the official kick-off to my fifty-plus-year music career.

I enjoyed the notoriety I received after the cultural evening. For the first time since starting at St Enda's, I felt I was worth something instead of constantly being berated and told how useless I was. The cultural evening also showed me there was life outside of my ridiculous situation in St. Enda's. After school, I began to hang out in town and develop friendships outside those six-foot walls. I was always the shy person in our friend group, but now I had something to look forward to each day after the darkness of school. I felt like I was living in two different worlds—the utter bizarreness of St. Enda's and the normalcy of hanging out with friends from other schools in town.

The Conversation

Mam sat me down just before my sixteenth birthday and asked what I would like as a gift, but also the bigger question of what I was thinking of doing after high school. Without hesitation, I said I wanted to be a professional musician and I'd love to get an electric guitar for my birthday. She didn't bat an eyelid when she said with a smile on her face, "Years ago, Seamus, I had a fortune teller say to me I would have a son whose name would be in lights someday." She quickly added that I had picked a profession where it was incredibly difficult to succeed.

That night I heard Mam talking to Dad in their bedroom adjacent to mine. I couldn't make out what they were saying, but I knew the electric guitar and, more importantly, my dream of becoming a professional musician were on the agenda. In the Irish household, you didn't talk to your father about career decisions. The vast majority of communication was done through your mother.

The next day, I was extremely nervous as I sat down after school with Mam for our daily cuppa tea and her delicious brown bread. The United Nations has no idea how to achieve world peace. Only the Irish understand that in every situation, no matter how dire, everyone should just sit back and have the cuppa tea and everything would be fine.

Mam said she talked to Dad and that they would support my dream of being a professional musician in any way they could, but on one condition. I had to finish my high school education first. I was shocked by the words that came out of her mouth. When I asked Mam what Dad's reaction was when she mentioned me becoming a professional musician, she said he replied, "Seamus has been at that feckin' thing (the guitar) day and night.

He seems to be good at it. How can we argue or get in the way of that kind of dedication?" From that day forward, their support for me and my dream never wavered. In the Ireland of 1970, the idea of someone making a living playing music, especially with the wild rock music I loved, must have seemed ludicrous. But Mam and Dad were forward-looking parents in so many ways.

Having to finish high school presented a bit of a problem. Since I picked up the guitar, I could not focus on schoolwork. But my parents had given me a lifeline, so I went about trying to catch up so I could at least scrape by until graduation which was still a few years off.

I struggled with reading from an early age. I could read the words on a page but couldn't connect the sentences in my head. It often took ten to fifteen minutes to read one page. Jane Austin's Persuasion was required reading for the Leaving Certificate—the state examination that determined graduation from high school and eligibility for college. I loved Jane Austin and the beautiful pictures she created with her extraordinary writing, but it took me over a year to make my way through the book. Things were further complicated by my inability to speak Gaelic well. All subjects at St. Enda's, even science, were taught through Gaelic making it almost impossible for me to learn. But now I had an end goal. I spent three hours a night at homework trying to catch up. It cut into my guitar time but I figured the tradeoff was worth it.

Shortly after my conversation with Mam, I got my electric guitar. Even before "the conversation," I picked it out and put it on hold at Raftery's with my buddy Mike McMahon. When I got home with the new bright red and white guitar, I figured out a way to put the needle arm of the record player on the headstock (top) of the guitar. By doing so and turning up the volume of the player to 10, I got a faint distorted guitar sound. To me it was a Marshall stack amplifier. I spent hours figuring out ingenious ways to tape the needle to the guitar. After a few weeks of destroying the record player and doing severe damage to our record collection in the process, I told Dad I needed an amplifier and a speaker for the electric guitar.

Dad was a skilled carpenter and very handy with electronics. He excused me from school one wet and windy afternoon. We went into town and set about going to the electronics and hardware stores to pick up the bits and pieces to construct an amplifier and speaker cabinet. I revered my dad, but we didn't do too many things together, partly because I spent so much time practicing guitar, but also because at that age, most teenagers didn't interact with their dads that much. I was beyond excited as we picked out the speaker, the wood for the speaker cabinet, and the glossy cloth to go over the speaker.

I stayed up late that night with Dad as he put the amp and the speaker cabinet together. It was a daunting task even for him, as the speaker cabinet had all kinds of unique specifications, and he didn't have the sophisticated tools normally used for that job. But he was determined to do it right and worked late into the evening making sure it was perfect. I'll never forget the moment I plugged my new shiny electric guitar into that amplifier. It was a few minutes after midnight and the house reeked from the smell of the black paint on the speaker cabinet. Dad just smiled; he saw the excitement on my face and the delight in my eyes when I hit my first power chord. He may as well have given me a brand-new sports car. I barely slept that night. I couldn't wait to crank the amplifier. Dad was always my hero, but when he finished putting the last screw into that amplifier, he was forever on a high pedestal in my mind.

After that night, all the emotions and frustrations that had built up inside from the bullshit at St. Enda's and my social isolation were poured into the guitar. I played day and night, keeping the whole family awake and haunting the neighbors. For a brief period, I felt in some ways normal. I was getting by at St. Enda's, I had some good friends and I had found my calling. Things were looking up—or so I thought.

A Time of Fear

The tranquility didn't last too long. The six northern-most counties of Ireland were under British rule and collectively referred to as the North. The population consisted of Catholics and Protestants. The Catholics had been discriminated against over the years, especially in the areas of housing and job opportunities. The predominantly Protestant population were commonly referred to as Loyalists because of their loyalty to the British Crown. The Catholic population, often called Nationalists, aspired to be part of the South in a United Ireland.

What started out as a series of peaceful civil rights marches in 1968 quickly descended into chaotic violence. In the space of a year, neighbors in Belfast, Derry and other cities and towns in the North, who once vacationed and sang songs together in Salthill, or at least co-existed in their neighborhoods, were engulfed in sectarian violence that lasted almost 30 years. The arrival of the British army in August of 1969 only made things worse. The daily images on television of armored cars, tanks and soldiers in full riot gear on Irish soil, engaged in running battles with the civilian population, were terrifying. The atrocities on all sides deeply affected me. I was saddened to see people who often followed the same football teams, ate the same food and listened to the same music, engage in such gruesome violence. It was heartbreaking to see the sadness in the eyes of all these people who looked exactly like me. When the nightly news came on television at 6:15 pm, I felt a deep sense of dread and anxiety.

On a summer's morning in 1969, I came down to the kitchen to find Mam crying. Dad had been called up as part of the army reserve. After serving in the army in WW II, Dad went on annual army training sessions that lasted several weeks. He loved that time as he got to meet those he served with during the war. I'm sure he also enjoyed the break from all of us. This time was different. In 1969, there was a palpable fear that full-scale civil war was about to break out in the North of Ireland and potentially spread to the South. Dad was put on active duty at age 53. Within a few days he was deployed as an army captain.

That was a difficult summer for all of us, but especially for Mam, who worried about Dad and all of us if the violence spread. In addition, we had a bed & breakfast business with up to ten guests on a given night throughout the summer months. Some or the guest were "full board" which meant, in addition to breakfast, they also had a midday and evening meal. Between taking care of five teenagers and catering to our guests, Mam was run off her feet. The girls were a great help to her during that time while I, on the other hand, managed to escape much of the work playing guitar or pitch and putt (par three golf) on a course across the street from where we lived.

Thankfully, the violence in the North didn't spread to the rest of Ireland and, after several months, Dad returned from deployment. Things were very difficult financially for Mam and Dad, partly because of the lost income during Dad's time in the reserve and partly because of the cost of raising a young family.

Changes

The following January, we gave up the B&B business. Mam went back to nursing after being away from it for over twenty years. In order to do that, she had to take an arduous course to be re-certified. She worked night duty in Merlin Park, a hospital on the outskirts of Galway. She was assigned to the geriatric ward doing three twelve-hour shifts one week and four the next. It was exhausting work with a lot of heavy lifting involved. As always, she never complained and talked lovingly about her patients and all the hospital staff. She was proud of her work and took my sister Ger and her boyfriend Enda up to meet some patients and the staff.

Around the time Mam went back to work, Dad started working as a taxi driver for a company called Big O Taxis. Within a short time, he decided to form Corrib Co-Op Cabs, one of the first co-ops of its kind in Ireland. When he was not driving, he manned the taxi office radio for hours on end and conducted meetings with the staff. He was also the Galway rep for the Taximen's Association. The taxi business suited him in many ways as he had an entrepreneurial spirit and was constantly coming up with new ideas to move the business forward. Dad loved meeting people and came home with hilarious stories about the passengers he had on his taxi runs.

As we started the 1970s, our family life was hectic as we were all on different schedules. My sisters were working or at college, and I was playing music and doing the part-time bar work. The only stipulation was that everyone had to be home for Sunday dinner. The rest of the week, schedules forced us to become fiercely independent. We had our own "text messaging" system in the form of a small writing pad near the stove in the kitchen, where we left messages for each other. They were simple things like, "Dad, dinner is on a plate in the fridge ready for the oven, 350 degrees for 20 minutes" or "Mam, do you know where my navy-blue shirt is?" Dad's notes were the best. A typical one would say, "Gone on run to Mullingar, back late, don't worry about dinner, dog and cat fed."

The First Fifteen Minutes

In the early 1970s, music continued to be the focus of my life. The long hours of practice were paying off. Damien and I played a lot together and eventually we got together with a drummer P.J. Duggan who played with St. Patrick's Brass Band in town, and a singer Mike Cazabon. One afternoon we sat in Cazabon's house chatting about music and singing a few songs. Then and there, we decided to form a group called Spoonful. The name came from a song from the band Cream.

Cazabon's family was originally from Trinidad. They were the first black family I remember in Galway growing up. Their mom was the salt of the earth and their dad, a doctor, was a big man who only came over from England where he worked a few times a year. Those visits were often documented by the arrival of another little Cazabon within months of the dad's departure. Like ours, the Cabazon household was a meeting place for all, and there was always a welcome and a spot at their table.

For no particular reason, I was assigned the role of lead guitar with Spoonful. I had to learn that skill quickly. There was a song by Creedence Clearwater Revival "Green River" in the jukebox at a local amusement hall. It had a simple guitar solo so I figured it was a good place to start. I played the song so many times that John Carney, the manager and cashier at the Casino, took it out of the jukebox and gave it to me. It was driving him crazy and he knew I wanted it. I had paid for it twenty times over.

Spoonful rehearsed every Sunday in a shed at the back of the drummer's house in Bohermore, a beautiful section of old Galway with tiny row houses. We had one small amplifier that we all played through, but we could be heard all over town. After a while, we migrated to an old building overlooking the Corrib River that weaves its way through Galway. It was a five-story walk-up on stairs that should have been condemned. The floorboards and rickety railings felt like they were about to give way every time we walked up the steep stairs. There was a constant moldy-smelling dampness in the air, and the water rushing down the Corrib in all its fury was deafening. But it was our space, our Abbey Road, and we each had access to the key which was hidden behind a stone at the top of the stairs. The 230 volts of power needed for our amplifiers came from a single light bulb socket, a fire hazard that we never considered for a minute—one's mortality is not top of mind at age 17. We practiced several days a week and developed a repertoire that consisted of "Sunshine of Your Love" and "Spoonful" from Cream along with some songs from the bands Ten Years After and Steppenwolf.

I never had much luck with the girls and saw myself as awkward and shy. There was a lovely girl who spent hours on the fifth floor of our rehearsal space listening to us practice. She had beautiful long flowing red hair and often wore a green summer dress with floral designs. She loved music and was constantly bopping along to the beat. She seemed to like the lead guitar as many days she stayed long after the band left to hear me practice. It never struck me for a moment that she might have fancied me, and I'm sure she didn't, but I was constantly teased about Mary by the band. The same girl, Mary Coughlan, went on to become an internationally renowned jazz singer, as beautiful today as she was then. Mary told me recently she once asked someone in Spoonful if she could sing a song with us and was abruptly put in her place for even suggesting it. Thankfully, it wasn't me who denied one of the world's great jazz singers an opportunity to sing with our band.

Our first gig was a "Young You" talent competition in Galway. The event was held in a small community center in the center of the beautiful Claddagh neighborhood in the heart of Galway. We selected three songs for our performance: "Proud Mary," "Spoonful," and "Love Like a Man." Mam and my sisters helped select my outfit for the show, an orange tie-die t-shirt with pieces of white wool Mam had sewn on the sleeves and blue bellbottom jeans. I had hair down to my shoulders and weighed in at 125 pounds soaking wet.

Playing the electric guitar for the first time to a big audience was exhilarating. I found something I loved to do, and I was as good or better at it than most anyone else, at least in the small town of Galway. I had that same tingling sensation I had performing at the cultural evening with Damien a few years earlier, but there was something viscerally different about playing the electric guitar. It felt like an extension of my body. From the moment I stepped on stage until we finished the last note, I was transported to another world, another planet. I felt every note rushing through my veins. It was a high like no other.

We won the talent competition and the day after the show, Mam and my sisters were walking down a laneway in Salthill to Sunday mass. A few local lads were walking ahead of them and much to Mam's amusement, one guy said, "Jesus fuckin' Christ, I was down at the fuckin' Claddagh Hall last night and there was a long-haired fuckin' weirdo who could make the fuckin' guitar talk." For the longest time after that, I became affectionately known to my friends as the long-haired fuckin' weirdo. It should be said, in Ireland, the F word is often used as an adjective to express emotion, although the young fellas in the laneway took it to an extreme.

After the competition, our photo appeared in the local Galway paper, the *Connaught Centennial*. This was bigger than the cultural evening. It was my first brush with fame—my first "fifteen minutes."

Soon after that, we started doing gigs at the Galway Tennis Club, where the youth of Galway gathered for bi-weekly "hops" or dances. Spoonful was now using multiple amplifiers, some of which were huge. Dad and some of his Corrib Co-Op taxi drivers were commandeered to transport the "gear" to the gigs. I'm sure the money came out of Dad's pocket; it was another example of him supporting my dream but always doing so in his quiet way.

Spoonful continued to gain popularity around Galway. It was good for me in many ways, but, in particular, on a social level. We had a wonderful following and I made some great friends, both male and female. There was also a great camaraderie within the band. We even had a manager, Romano Magliocco, whose parents came from Italy. He was a little older than us, very handsome and a dapper dresser. He had a great way about him and perfect for the role of band manager.

Despite all the buzz with Spoonful, I was hearing a different kind of music. Rory Gallagher, the legendary Irish blues guitar player, was having a huge influence on me, as was Jimi Hendrix, B.B. King and Eric Clapton, and I was eager to try something new. The pop music of Spoonful and some of the band's limitations made me decide to move on in late 1971. It was hard to leave the band less than a year after it started. I left Spoonful on the best of terms. They knew I was moving in a different direction with my music.

I don't think I was fully prepared for life without Spoonful. I felt very alone and unsure of what was next. I missed the increasing notoriety I got during my tenure with the band. I also missed the daily interactions with the guys. I questioned my decision as I saw the band do very well without me.

Several months after leaving Spoonful, I started playing with a gifted organ player, Sean O'Healy, and a fine drummer, Martin Commins. We formed a new band called Life's Feast, a name we took from Shakespeare's Macbeth that means the good things in life. The music was very different. From day one, we did our own thing. It was probably the most honest period of my early musical career. The music was experimental and at least half of our set list was original material. Life's Feast did some exciting and different shows around Galway. After a year, the band began to fade, but I treasure those moments of musical exploration.

The Clouds

By late 1972, I knew things weren't right with me. I was feeling down a lot of the time. I couldn't understand why people were smiling and laughing when there was nothing to laugh or smile about. I was terrified and distressed by the continuing violence in the North. I was overwhelmed by an incredible feeling of sadness and anxiety and lost all hope for the future. I still loved the music but found little joy in anything else.

One night after a dance, I was walking home through the streets of Galway when I was jumped by a bunch of drunk teenagers. They knocked me to the ground and kicked me, aiming for my head and stomach. Eventually someone recognized me and said, "That's fuckin' Seamy Kelleher, the guitar guy; leave him alone." The guy helped me up and apologized for the beating doled out by his buddies. But the damage was done. I do believe it was a random act of drunkenness, but I was in a fragile state before the beating and the violence of that attack stayed with me day and night for months afterwards and became a sort of paranoia in my mind. I was afraid to go out on my own and was constantly looking over my shoulder to see if someone was following me. I was shaken to the core.

Despite my deteriorating mental condition, I did manage to scrape by my Leaving Certificate Examination in 1972. I found out forty-five years later Mam paid one of my best friends, Brendan Mahon, five pounds ($15 at the time) to tutor me in math just before the exam. I had no idea I was being tutored—I just thought we were studying together.

Mam and Dad were incredibly relieved I passed the Leaving Certificate. They both placed great value in an education. Dad insisted that each of my sisters have some kind of skill beyond the Leaving Cert that would provide them independence. He had seen enough Irish women end up in abusive situations because they depended on their husbands for an income.

Shortly after the Leaving Cert, I went back to school at the newly opened College of Technology in Galway. I figured I'd give Electronic Engineering a try as it would help me with my amplifiers and electric guitars. The college was a wonderful bright and airy place. I couldn't believe that you didn't have to be in prison with a bunch of miserable bastards walking around the halls with leather straps in order to get an education. More and more, I began to resent those wasted years in St. Enda's.

As good as the environment was at the College of Technology, after a month or so, I knew it wasn't working for me. Each day sitting in class, all I could hear were heavy guitar riffs going through my head along with a pounding bass and drums. My fingers were constantly in motion shaping guitar chords and solos. The lecturer's voice felt like it was in the distant background. But I was determined to stick it out.

Skull and Thin Lizzy

I started a new band, Skull, with Dave Cazabon, the younger brother of Mike, the lead singer with Spoonful. The drummer was Frankie Mulveen. Frankie had long straight blond hair and traveled around Galway on an Easy-Rider style motorcycle complete with the high handlebars. Cazabon was a smaller version of Jimi Hendrix and in some ways just as wild. He had an afro and, like Frankie, could be seen driving around town like a lunatic on his green Honda 175 motorcycle. I wasn't quite as cool as Frankie and Dave. My mode of transportation was a red and white Honda 50 scooter with a top speed of 50 mph. To make matters worse, I had a huge helmet that made my tiny body seem completely out of proportion.

Dave and Frankie were simply crazy and seemed to live on the edge. I was the quiet one in the band but once on stage, we had that elusive chemistry and that's where the wild side of me came out. It was not unusual for my guitar to get launched across the stage. It was my way of expressing myself. I was very conscious of my stage image and often performed in high platform boots, blue jeans, and a black vest with nothing underneath. Dave and Frankie were equally stage conscious paying attention to every detail of their clothing. Our shows were a feast for the eyes. I bought some stage lights to make things even more visually appealing.

I didn't drink or take any drugs, so it fell to me to run every aspect of the band from the equipment to the bookings and organizing the music. As the months wore on, I did little or no schoolwork at the College of Technology and still couldn't tell AC from DC power despite multiple electrical engineering courses.

I got a call one day from a booking agent in Galway who hired bands for the many venues around town. He asked if Skull would be interested in opening for an up-and-coming band from Dublin called Thin Lizzy. I was already familiar with some of their music and loved it, so I immediately said yes. We agreed on a fee of seven pounds—to be split between the three members of the band. We were basically paying to play. Two weeks later, we were on stage at the Hanger Ballroom, a few hundred yards from my house, opening for Thin Lizzy. With over 700 people at the show, there was an air of excitement as word on the street was this band from Dublin was going places.

Thin Lizzy was a three-piece band at that time with Phil Lynott on vocals and bass, Brian Downey on drums and Eric Bell on lead guitar. Phil's dad was from British Guiana and his mom from Dublin. He was over six-foot tall with an exotic afro hairstyle reminiscent of Jimi Hendrix—total rock star material. Before Thin Lizzy took the stage, Phil thanked us for opening up and said he really enjoyed our set. He was beyond kind to us as were the other band members. A few months later, Lizzy came back to town and requested we open for them again. This time around, there were well over a thousand people crammed into the Hanger Ballroom to hear them. The place was buzzing as Lizzy were getting increasingly popular all over Ireland. It was nerve racking to be on stage in front of that many people. As we finished our set, the roadie called me over to the side of the stage and said Thin Lizzy were delayed getting to Galway, and we would have to extend our show. That meant repeating some songs with extended guitar solos and doing other songs we had never done before. We stepped things up and the audience responded. After we finished, Thin Lizzy were incredibly apologetic for being late. Once again, they were a pleasure to hang out with and just chat. There was marijuana and other drugs in abundance being offered to everyone in the dressing room, but I didn't partake as I was just interested in the music. Thin Lizzy and crew found it amusing that Skull was a three-piece rock band that happened to have a black bass player with an afro who was obsessed with Phil Lynott and Jimi Hendrix.

A few weeks after the show at the Hanger, I heard a song on the radio that put my hair on end. It was an old Irish ballad song "Whiskey in the Jar." But it was done with a rock beat and there was a hauntingly beautiful lead guitar playing all the way through it. It was Thin Lizzy and within a few weeks, the song was near the top of the British Charts, a first for an Irish rock band.

I got a call from the booking agent asking if Skull would open up for Thin Lizzy at a big ballroom called Talk of the Town. Interestingly, the fee was still seven pounds, despite the success of Thin Lizzy and I'm sure a big increase in the agent's booking fee. On the night of the show, things were different. The amplification system was massive and there were all kinds of lights around the stage. The road crew had expanded dramatically and they treated us like crap. The head roadie told me we could no longer use any of the band's gear. I responded saying I didn't have our equipment with me and it wouldn't be enough to fill the venue even if I had. He called Thin Lizzy at their hotel and Phil Lynott got on the phone and said, "Those guys have been with us for the past year, they can use all of our fuckin' stuff, even the guitars if they want to." Suddenly, the roadies changed their tune and gave us everything we needed for the show.

There were over 2000 people at the Talk of the Town that evening. I looked out at the mass of people and wondered what it would be like to have that kind of crowd every night. The audience responded well to our music, but they were there to hear Thin Lizzy and Ireland's new anthem,

45

"Whiskey in the Jar." It was still an extraordinary experience for a young three-piece band from Galway to open for a national act.

I was impressed by Thin Lizzy that night but figured it was only a matter of time before our day in the spotlight would come. Galway was a small town of twenty-five thousand people, so it was safe to say most people my age were at the show. It gave Skull and me great visibility around town.

After the show, the booking agent disappeared without paying us our seven pounds. I went straight to Phil Lynott and explained the situation. He said in his heavy Dublin accent, "Seamy, come down to the Imperial Hotel in the morning and we'll straighten things out."

The next morning, I arrived at the hotel just as Thin Lizzy were getting ready to hit the road for their next show. Their new-found popularity was evident by throngs of people in the lobby of the hotel vying for the band's attention. I locked eyes with Phil once I walked in the door and he came straight over to me. Without blinking, he pulled out a wad of money and peeled off the money I was owed. He apologized for the way I was treated by the agent and roadies. He said, "Seamy, let's get the fuck out of here so I can buy you a drink."

I had an important decision to make and it had to be quick. I had to find the bar in Galway where the most people could see me hanging out with Phil Lynott from Thin Lizzy. There was only one place to go, the Cellar Bar on Eglinton Street. The Cellar was where all the hip people gathered on Saturday mornings to recover from the previous night's hangovers. They were Galway's professional elite cool people—the special forces of drinking. Heads turned when this newly minted bona fide six-foot one Irish rock star from Dublin walked in with this skinny little local guy. I ordered an orange juice while Phil had a perfect pint from the wide-eyed bartender. I have zero memory of what we talked about but I clearly recall walking back to the Imperial Hotel with my friend Phil and my head getting bigger with every stride.

The next time I saw Phil Lynott was three years later in 1976 at Madison Square Garden when Thin Lizzy shared the bill with Queen. Sadly, we lost Phil in 1986 to an illness brought on by drug addiction. I'll never forget his kindness to a little band from Galway called Skull. He set the bar high for how I should treat musicians throughout my career and I've done my best to honor his kindness and example at every turn.

My second fifteen-minute brush with fame as the opening act for Thin Lizzy didn't go to my head for too long as I continued to work in the Oslo in Salthill and in a bar in the center of Galway called the Genoa, which was run by the Magliocco family. The owner, Mr. Magliocco, was a tough boss but he treated me very well. I worked at the Genoa and the Oslo several days a week, which provided me with the money to buy my guitars and amps—and fund my friends' drinking, which I was happy to do.

The sadness I started feeling when I finished my Leaving Certificate stayed with me. Some days were worse than others. I went for several weeks at a time feeling relatively normal; then without any warning or apparent cause, I fell into complete darkness. I hid what was happening from my family and friends. Despite my struggles, I have fond memories of going to concerts and just hanging out with friends during the good periods.

After less than a year in college, I knew I was going nowhere in terms of academia. I asked my mechanics teacher why I got 10% on one of my exams. Without hesitation he said, "Seamus, that's because you're a nice young man and managed to spell your name correctly." We both laughed heartily knowing it was time for me to end my college experience, at least for the time being.

Saved by the Bell

Through a contact of Dad, I got a job at Standard Pressed Steel International (SPS), a large factory on the outskirts of Galway making nuts and bolts for American cars. It was a grueling and dangerous job, but Ireland was in a deep recession and jobs were scarce. The factory was a dark dreary place without any natural light. I worked on large machines where massive coils of steel were fed into presses and forged into nuts and bolts. It was backbreaking work where all day long, I was lifting a ten-pound sledgehammer over my shoulder replacing die casts in the presses. The machines were lubricated with filthy recycled oil due to a worldwide oil shortage. Within a few months, my hands were ripped apart by tiny shards of steel flying from the filthy machines. Each day after work, I used a needle from Mam's sewing machine to pry the metal from my fingers. Several workers on the factory floor were missing fingers or had damaged arms and legs due to accidents on the factory floor.

What made the work bearable were my co-workers from every corner of Galway County. It was my first real exposure to people beyond the Galway City area. I enjoyed the interaction and even the teasing I got as the city boy not used to the grueling work. Many of them went home after a twelve-hour shift and worked on the family farm for several hours. They were protective of me and made sure I was as safe as I could be, given the environment. I worked the day shift one week and nights the next. The nights were hard as I went to work when my friends were hanging out in the bars or going to concerts and dances.

Despite opening up for Thin Lizzy and the many fun shows that followed, my band Skull had come to an end and I wondered if I would ever get back to the music. I still practiced for hours each day, but the dream of performing professionally was fading fast.

Between the factory and bartending at the Oslo and Genoa, I was putting in at least sixty hours a week. There was no need for me to work that hard. It had nothing to do with money as I had a healthy savings account. I was trying to keep busy to mask the darkness in my head which was getting worse by the day.

I was on the factory floor swinging the sledgehammer one afternoon when the foreman, a rough and ready taskmaster, came up to me and said, "Kelleher, there are some lads here to see you." Instead of bringing me to the office away from the noise and the danger posed by the horrible pressing machines, he brought the visitors over to my workspace. Nobody should have been on the factory floor without protective gear, especially in the area where I was.

My co-workers looked my way as one of the visitors was a well-known musician Ja Reedy from a popular band the Philosophers. The other was a local singer Liam Merrigan who, because of his extraordinary voice, was making a name for himself around town with various bands. Ja wore a black leather jacket and had that rock star aura about him with his slick-backed hair. Liam was an imposing figure with an Elvis haircut complete with sideburns.

Ja got straight to the point saying, "Seamus, we want you to join our new band Rock & Roll Circus." It was the last thing I expected to hear. I didn't know what to say. I had given up on the idea of making a living with music, but told Ja and Liam I would think about it. After they left, I picked up the sledgehammer but couldn't focus on work for the remainder of my shift. I'm lucky I didn't kill myself that day as all I could think of was playing music on stage with a new band made up of some of Galway's finest musicians. My mind was racing as I left the factory and drove home on my Honda 50. Part of me wanted to jump at the chance to escape the dreadful conditions of SPS and join these amazing musicians on a great adventure, but I wasn't sure if I was good enough to play in a band with them. I also worried what my parents would think of me leaving a steady job.

I told my Mam and Dad that night, almost in passing, what happened on the factory floor. I know they were still hoping I would go back to school, but based on my performance at the College of Technology, they knew I wasn't ready. They worried about my physical health and could see I was incredibly sad all the time. My hands were badly infected from the steel shards and I was breaking out in a red rash all over my body from the recycled oil. Each night, Mam washed my blue uniform with a paint thinner in a futile attempt to get the entrenched black oil stains out. No matter how hard I scrubbed my body, I couldn't get the oil off my skin. The stains were a constant reminder the job was taking a toll on mind and body.

Two days after telling my parents about the job offer, Mam came to me and said, "Seamus, I talked to Dad and we think you should consider taking the job with the band. We're worried about your health. You don't need to be working under those awful conditions at SPS. We know you love the music and that's where your heart is, and we will always support you." My jaw dropped. Instantly, I felt a huge weight off my chest. I went up to my room and cried tears of joy. I tried so hard to be a success in college but failed miserably. Despite my best efforts, I knew I was no good at the factory job. I felt I had let my parents down even though they never saw it that way. The emotions I held inside for many months were flowing. But now there was hope.

Joining the Circus

I gave two weeks' notice at the factory and started rehearsing with Ja, Liam, and Andy McEntee, a local Galway drummer. Ja was the most naturally talented musician I ever played with and an incredibly hard worker. He also had the ability to drink incredible amounts of Guinness and still be the same person but just funnier. I never saw him drunk or abusive to anybody. Liam Merrigan didn't drink but was as quirky as the day was long. Despite being a chain smoker, his voice came directly from the heavens. It was a cross between Elvis Presley, Roy Orbison and the Everly Brothers, only better than all of them. Andy was a great drummer, and like the other members of the band, a hard worker. He was married with two children and struggled financially, as everyone in the band did except for me. I was still bar tending in the Oslo and Genoa and had no expenses to speak of.

Within a short time, Andy and I became great friends and spent many a day in his flat eating slices of toast with raspberry jam, discussing the woes of the band. The bread was cheap because Andy worked for a local bakery. It was fine, as we were 100 percent confident we were going to make it big with the Circus. We were the "dreamers of dreams," to quote the poet Arthur O'Shaughnessy.

I felt way out of my league with the band, especially in the early days. Ja, Liam and Andy were several years older than me and well-seasoned musicians. They were incredibly patient and gave me the time to develop the basic skills I lacked. Before joining the band, I had set only one condition: that I be allowed play the theme song from the then-popular TV show Hawaii Five-O. I'm sure Ja and Billy wondered if they were making the right decision since I didn't ask for more money or anything. At the conclusion of our final rehearsal before we launched the band, I said, "What about Hawaii Five-O?" Ja and Liam rolled their eyes but said okay. I put together this crazy arrangement of the TV theme complete with key modulations, police sirens and explosions using the latest technology available. It took a few times around to get everything the way I wanted it, but I knew instantly Hawaii Five-O was going to be fun to do live. Ja and Bill had delivered on their promise, so I was happy.

We did our first show at the Ocean Wave in Salthill, one of the many new cabaret venues opening in the area. These venues were different from the traditional ballrooms where people were focused on dancing and only soft drinks and sandwiches were available at the bar. The reverse was the case at the Ocean Wave where people sat at tables and alcohol was served. The audience expected to be entertained—they wanted a show—we didn't disappoint.

From the moment we started, there was a great response from the audience. We were different from the other bands around town that were mostly doing the same songs night after night. We had Liam Merrigan—or Elvis as Andy and I started referring to him—Andy's energetic drumming, and my out-of-control guitar playing, while Ja's harmonies took Liam's voice places it had never been before. At one point in the evening, I looked over at Ja and mouthed Hawaii Five-0. I could tell he was reluctant to risk what so far had been a great launch for the band. But good to his word, he announced the song. The audience seemed a bit perplexed as they hadn't heard Hawaii Five-0 other than on the TV show, and they certainly had never heard it played on the electric guitar. After a few minutes, everyone looked up at the stage. By the time the song finished, the place erupted in applause and cheering, a reaction that was highly unusual for a local

Galway band. I was thrilled with myself but was embarrassed by the attention turning every color of red. Ja, Liam and Andy were all smiles. They knew they had made the right decision going with the clueless nineteen-year-old, wildly immature and innocent guitar player.

Initially, the gigs were in small pubs. We were paid 20 pounds a night and that was for the whole band. One of the early gigs was in a bar called the Forge in Tuam, a small town twenty miles from Galway. The bar was perfectly set up for music with a large seating area focused on the stage. Within weeks, we were getting several encores. Monday was an off night for most musicians, so they came to the Forge in Tuam to hear this crazy band from Galway. The place was full of colorful characters and we were never short of talented guest artists who wanted to join the Circus for at least one night. Those Monday nights were some of the most memorable shows I've ever played.

Playing pubs and the cabaret spots all over Galway, we quickly developed a large following of all ages. There was a definite buzz about the band. By the autumn of '73 we were expanding to the small towns around County Galway. Our sound system was getting bigger and we had a number of the same people following us for each show. Hawaii Five-0 became the crowd favorite and we often played it twice or even three times a night. I was in my element.

There are no words to describe what it's like to be part of a band that strikes a chord with the public. Each night, you see the crowds growing with new faces being exposed to your music. It's an intoxicating experience and probably explains why so many musicians keep chasing their dreams despite the financial hardships, failure and rejection that is part and parcel of the business.

Love Strikes

It was the spring of '73 when I met Mary. She was attending college in Galway. I had just started working with Rock & Roll Circus after leaving the factory job. Mary was a beautiful girl with long straight fair hair. She was no more than five feet tall, but she had a larger-than-life spirit and a wonderful smile that always caused my heart to miss a beat or two.

Mary was my first girlfriend. As I got ready to go on our first date, my sisters were helping me pick out what to wear. They asked me her last name but I didn't know it, so I said, "Mary Thing." The name stuck and that's what I called her and it's still what comes to mind when I think of her.

We had a beautiful relationship spending many hours just walking around Galway and going for rides on my Honda 50 scooter. On Sunday afternoons we took trips along the Atlantic coast to the wilds of Connemara and up by the beautiful river Corrib. We had a lot of mutual friends so most evenings we met up in the pubs around Galway. After the pubs closed, we spent the nights and early morning chatting together in a flat she shared with two girlfriends. We fell in love and while my mood continued to be dark most days, there were many happy times with Mary and her friends. My family was amused and I'm sure happy to see me in a relationship, since up to that point, the guitar had always been my one and only interest.

By the fall of '73, Rock & Roll Circus was gaining traction. Ja and Liam signed a management contract with Hugh Hardy, a high-profile figure in the Irish music scene. Hardy wanted to turn Liam into an Elvis impersonator. That was a mistake since Liam was just as talented singing a whole range of songs. He was also on the heavy side and did not exactly exude the sexuality from the stage that Hardy had in mind. Setting him up as the next Elvis was inviting failure for Liam and, indeed, the rest of the band. Up until that point, it was a band devoid of egos. We all had our strong points. Despite my early insecurities with the band, after a few months my guitar playing was on equal footing with Liam's amazing voice. Under the new arrangement, everything changed. It was the beginning of the end of a great band.

Liam is the Gaelic for William (Bill), so to put Liam front and center, Hardy changed the name of the band to Billy Kid and the Pirates, although I continued to call the band Rock & Roll Circus. He suggested we add a keyboard player. The guy we picked was a prodigy musician, incredibly bright and very funny, but the addition of keyboards took the rawness out of the band. We lost our unique sound, a sound that doesn't come around too often, if at all, in the life of a musician.

Hardy tried to convince us we would become stars with this new sound, but I knew the success we had worked so hard to achieve was being ripped out of our hands. I found it hard to take but held on to the hope that the band might still be a launching pad for my career.

We recorded Elvis Presley's hits "Heartbreak Hotel" and "Jailhouse Rock" in one of Dublin's top recording studios. It should have been an incredibly exciting experience for me as it was my first time in a recording studio, but I was feeling very low and increasingly anxious as the day progressed. While the recording sounded okay, there was nothing original or special about it and a far cry from the music we had been playing just a few months earlier as a four-piece band. Hardy also used another drummer from Galway for the recording session which was hard for Andy, and it also sent a message to me that in Hardy's eyes, we were just the backing band or side men for "Elvis."

The record did get some airplay thanks to a big PR blitz from Hardy and soon we were on the road traveling the length and breadth of Ireland. To our followers in Galway, we were rock stars. Our tour bus, which Ja and Liam literally found in a junk yard, looked like the bus from The Partridge Family TV show, complete with bright yellow skylights. But in reality, it was a rundown heap of scrap, constantly breaking down, often in the middle of nowhere at three or four in the morning and in the cold, pouring rain.

We did six or seven shows a week in every corner of Ireland. The crowds were generally good as Hardy invested a lot of money in promoting the band. The audiences weren't sure what to make of us. We didn't fit the typical Irish showband mold. They were used to seven- or eight-piece showbands doing the latest pop and country hits. I felt sorry for Liam. Now the front man, the responsibility to make the show great fell solely on his shoulders. Promotion postcards were printed with an image of him in a white suit, without the band, looking like the Elvis heart throb from the 1950s. The postcard and what the audience saw on stage didn't match.

Heartbreak

I often brought my mother tea and brown bread early in the morning after coming back from the gigs with Rock & Roll Circus. One Monday, I got home earlier than expected from a show we did in Ballybunnion, County Kerry at the southernmost tip of Ireland. I decided 7 am was too early to bring Mam the cuppa tea. One of my sisters woke me a few hours later to tell me Mam died in her sleep. I was numb and didn't cry—I was in total disbelief. My biggest fear since I was a little boy became a reality that morning. Mam had a heart attack a year prior to her passing but she made a remarkable recovery and seemed in good health before her death. Her sudden passing was a shock to all of us.

Like us all, Mam had her flaws; she was not perfect. But I don't know if I've met a kinder person in my life. She has been gone well over forty years, but I still see that kindness in her eyes when I think of her. As the youngest and only male with four older sisters, Mam spoiled me but we had an amazing relationship that went deep. In the months before she passed, I'm thankful I got to spend a lot of time with her. Rock & Roll Circus was gaining momentum and most days, the band came to our house during the day to rehearse. Mam made sure she had fresh tea, brown bread and biscuits on hand during those long practice sessions. The best part of my day was sitting down with her for that cuppa tea. She was a great listener. I was able to tell her everything. I didn't just lose Mam that day; I lost a great friend and my biggest supporter.

Everything was a haze for me in the days following Mam's passing. I spent a lot of time with my good friend Brendan Glynn—one of those rare individuals who you can go for an hour-long walk with and not have to say a word if you don't need to. My girlfriend Mary was also very supportive and comforting during that time. There wasn't much to say; she knew I was traumatized by my loss.

I was more worried about Dad than anything. Like the rest of us, he depended on Mam for everything. My sisters and I couldn't imagine how he would manage without her. Mam was waked in the house. I remember Dad walking into their bedroom to say his final goodbye. As they took the body out of the house in the pine coffin with silver handles, he simply said, "I really loved Mary." The poor man was never the same after losing the love of his life.

Rock & Roll Circus had a big gig in Galway on the day my mother was buried. I asked Dad what I should do, and he answered, "What would Mam want you to do?" I had my answer but it was hard to play the show that night; my heart was broken into tiny pieces and I struggled through each song. I just wanted to cry. The idea that I would never sit down and have another cup of tea with Mam was devastating.

For the next several weeks, my sisters and I made sure Dad was never alone. He slept in my room as we wanted to change Mam and Dad's room around. We all found our own ways to cope with the loss. After a few weeks, Dad went back to the taxi rank. The girls and I were thankful he had some great friends in the business who kept a close eye on him.

The Breakdown

I didn't have time to mope around the house for long. I was back on the road six days a week. But I knew something wasn't right. The darkness and sadness I experienced intermittently over the past few years lasted for longer periods. I had a feeling of total hopelessness. I couldn't find any joy in life and was constantly sad. I spent as much time as possible sleeping as a way of coping with the mental anguish I experienced. The music, which normally brought relief, wasn't doing it anymore. My relationship with Mary was up and down as I withdrew into myself.

I did go see a doctor who said I was run down. She prescribed some kind of tonic. Depression, anxiety and stress were not even mentioned during my visit. Surely that should have been part of the conversation since the signs of mental illness were there in glaring clarity—she blew it.

My world came crashing down a week after the doctor's visit when we played a gig in Wexford on the east coast of Ireland, over a hundred miles from Galway. During the show, I had a hard time concentrating on the music. I was incredibly nervous, not about my performance, but about being able to finish the show. After the gig, I went back to the hotel. The band members were sitting around having a few drinks. That was always a fun time with storytelling and good-natured teasing, often at my expense since I was the youngest in the band. I told the guys I wasn't feeling great and went straight to bed. I couldn't fall asleep and got agitated to the point of panicking. I never experienced anything like that before. I got dressed, left the hotel and walked around the town at 5 am trying to shake it off. I banged on the doors of houses with shiny brass plaques outside indicating a doctor's office, in the hope that someone would hear me, but to no avail.

Eventually, I went back to the hotel and woke Ja. There was a worried look on his face and knew instantly something was terribly wrong. He had the hotel manager find a doctor willing to see me, no easy feat on a quiet Sunday morning in Ireland.

The doctor talked to me for close to an hour. He said he wasn't a psychiatrist but, in his opinion, I was suffering from depression and anxiety, and I was mentally and physically exhausted. My situation was most likely triggered by the recent loss of my mother. He reassured me I would be okay, but I needed professional help and it would take some time to recover.

I felt immediate relief just knowing that there was hope. The doctor gave me an injection that knocked me out for almost two days. The band had another show that Sunday night and performed without me after making sure there was someone to keep an eye on me at our hotel. They decided to get me back home early next morning before the sleep medication wore off.

In the Ireland of the 1970s, the church missions took place in the month of June. It was a time of renewal for Catholics. During the season, vending stalls were set up in church parking lots all over Ireland to sell religious artifacts such as statues of Jesus and Mary, rosary beads and every version of the holy cross imaginable.

Our tour bus was parked next to one of the mission stalls. I was half awake but severely medicated. Ja could see that things were going downhill quickly. He put me in the back of the bus hoping I'd sleep my way to Galway. Liam was driving and was without doubt the worst driver in Ireland. It was not unusual for him to overtake a truck or two on a blind corner of a tiny winding country road. When he took the wheel, we prepared to meet our Maker. It took Liam forever to get going out of the church parking lot and eventually Ja said, "Let's get the fuck out of here." All I remember next is the sight and sounds of breaking glass and wooden beams coming through the yellow skylights of our Partridge Family bus. Statues of Jesus crashed to the ground and rosary beads were strewn all over the top of the bus.

The entire stand was demolished. To make things worse, Liam was a God-fearing man. He didn't drink and never messed around with women. His only vice was the cigarettes, which perpetually hung from his mouth. One of the support beams from the mission stand was lodged in the skylight of the bus. Liam stopped to survey the damage. Not only had he severely damaged the bus, but in his mind, he had just committed the worst kind of sin by demolishing the stand and defacing all those religious symbols.

Ja got out of the bus, un-lodged the beam and said, "Let's go," but Liam wanted to stay and call the police. Ja said, "We need to get this kid back to Galway now." We pulled out of the parking lot with rosary beads still dangling from the roof of the bus. There was silence for a few minutes with everyone expecting to hear police sirens, but we didn't. Despite my dire situation, I began to smile and the rest of the band broke into howls of laughter. I found out years later that Hardy, our manager, was stuck with a hefty bill for the damages we caused—poetic justice for the damage he inflicted on our wonderful band.

After arriving back in Galway, I explained as best I could to Dad and my sisters what happened. Dad was already concerned about me being on the road because I was a terrible eater, but once Mam died, he worried even more as he knew she always had something on hand that I would eat.

After Mam passed, I had no appetite and was rapidly losing weight despite the "tonic" from the doctor.

I knew what I was feeling was terribly different than before. Previously, I got relief from the darkness at different times of the day. Now there was no relief and I experienced anxiety and panic attacks around the clock. Waking up in the morning was the hardest, having to face another day of hell. The thought of suicide crossed my mind. I just wanted the pain to end.

One night, I picked up a bread knife and put it to my wrist. I don't think I had any intention of hurting myself that evening, but it was a form of insurance if things got much worse. I worried about how my father and my sisters would be if I ended my life. They were just coming to grips with Mam's death. I couldn't add to the pain they were all experiencing but at the same time, I felt I was a burden on them. Would they be better off without me? I didn't know what to do. I was trapped.

A Wise Man

Dad called me aside a few days later and said, "Seamus, we need to get you some help. I don't think a regular doctor is what you need at this point. We have to find someone who knows something about how the brain works. You've been very nervous over the past year or so and constantly worrying about things you can't control. You need to start taking care of number one." He was surprised when I said, "Dad, if we don't do something now, I don't know how long I can last like this."

Dad said he had a friend at St Patrick's Psychiatric Hospital in Dublin who might be able to help me. St. Pat's, or the loony bin as we often referred to it as kids, was well known for alcoholism treatment and its expertise in depression and other mental illnesses. We knew people who had gone there, often in a bad way. Many recovered but some were never the same again.

The next day, Dad, my sister Maura and I drove up to St Pat's in Dublin. There's a great irony in that St. Pat's is located directly across from the Guinness Brewery—only in Ireland. The smell of burning yeast from the brewery was thick in the air before we even got out of the car. The lush hospital grounds were in stark contrast to the dark grey city of Dublin in the early 1970s.

After checking in, the three of us met Dad's friend Dr. Sugrue, the psychiatrist assigned to me. As she took my case history, she made it very clear that failing to give truthful answers to her questions would make it impossible for her to help me.

Over the course of two hours, I unloaded everything. I left nothing out. My sister Maura told me years later that it was one of the most difficult things she ever witnessed. Her heart broke hearing her young brother pouring out his feelings and watching Dad trying to take in what was coming out of my mouth. He was still in the midst of unimaginable grief after losing his wife only two months earlier, and now he heard his only son describe in excruciating detail the pain he had been going through for well over a year. I talked about the horrors of St. Enda's and the fear I was experiencing with the violence in the North of Ireland. Dad had no idea how bad things were in St. Enda's. I also described how alcohol abuse at home had caused me worry and pain.

At the end of the session, Dr. Sugrue confirmed I was suffering from reactive depression. It was building over a period of years, but the recent severity of it was likely triggered by the death on my mother. Like the good doctor in Dublin, she assured me I would recover but it would take time.

The doctor warned Dad and Maura I would be in hospital for at least three weeks. Dad was relieved knowing I was finally getting the help I desperately needed. I have absolutely no doubt that Dad's sixth sense and his wisdom, combined with the limitless love and support of my sisters, saved my life. The darkness I was dealing with was depression. It was a real thing and now there was a word for the darkness. Depression was something I'd have to learn to live with and manage for the rest of my life.

The Cuckoo's Nest

I don't remember too much about the first few weeks in St. Pat's, as most of the time was spent sleeping. My mind and body were exhausted from the mental and physical agitation I had been dealing with for so long, compounded by the trauma of losing Mam. However, I do have a clear memory of my first two days at St. Pat's as the medication I was taking hadn't fully kicked in. I ended up on a floor reserved for the most severe psychotic cases. When I think back, I see pictures in my mind of items flying across the hospital ward, patients being restrained by orderlies, and images of half-naked crazy people running around the place. Those memories have never left me to the point when I saw One Flew over the Cuckoo's Nest with Jack Nicholson a year later, it brought everything back to me in a disturbing and most vivid way. I still can't sit through the entire movie.

After a few days of utter madness, I was moved to another floor with young and old patients, all dealing with the hell and darkness that is depression and, for some, the curse of alcohol addiction.

Someone once asked me during one of my bad attacks to define depression. I remember my answer: "If you can come up with your worst vision of hell and multiply it by a thousand, then maybe you'll get a sense of how bad it is."

The new ward was small with less than forty people in all. I got to know my fellow patients relatively quickly. Some had been there for several weeks and were nearing the end of their treatment. Others were back for a second, third, or twentieth time. It was disturbing to think that this could very well be a lifelong affliction.

I met a lovely old man in St. Pat's, Mr. Duigan, from Donegal, and we became great friends. He suffered from recurrent depression—a type of depression that returned at regular intervals without warning, sometimes a few years apart but often just months between episodes. He was in and out of St Pat's for well over twenty years. He knew the institution well and the process that one went through from admission to discharge. He became my mentor.

Mr. Duigan and I had animated conversations in the mornings about politics, sports and music. The Nixon impeachment was taking place during our hospitalization and it was all over the television news. Just a few hours after our great and often funny conversations, Mr. Duigan would drift away and his silent suffering began. Even though he was still sitting next to me, it felt like he had gone to a faraway sad place. Watching him reminded me that my journey to the darkness was only a few hours away. At around 6 pm each day, my depression began and lasted most of the night.

There was another friend on the ward who was either animated and upbeat or very sad. He suffered from manic depression and the medical staff had a hard time getting him stable. At some point he received electroconvulsive therapy, the treatment of last resort for those struggling with deep depression. While it was successful with some patients, it had a devastating impact on others. The last time I saw my friend, he was sitting in a lounge chair staring out into space with a vacant look on his face. I lived in fear I might end up having to get electroconvulsive therapy if my depression failed to lift.

The hospital ward had its own clock. The highpoint of the day was the distribution of antidepressants and other medicines in the morning and evening. The rest of the day was spent managing your depression or addiction. There were seminars to explain what depression was and how you learn to live with it. I also had private meetings with my psychiatrist every few days.

After a week mostly spent in bed except for meals, my nurse told me I could go to the candy shop. The meds were doing their job and the therapy was working so I felt much better. I jumped out of bed, grabbed some money, and walked the five or six steps from the ward down a stairway to the shop. I got down the steps fine, but on the way back up, I went flat on my back with the candy splattered all over the floor. A week lying in bed, combined with the effects of the antidepressants and sleeping tablets, made my legs feel like rubber bands, incapable of supporting my body. My mouth felt like sandpaper, completely dry from the exertion of walking just a few steps. Prior to St Pat's, I had never taken anything more than an aspirin.

As the medical staff reduced the medication, I slowly emerged from my long sleep and the accompanying haze. I stayed up for longer periods, gradually increasing the time I was able to stay awake. The depression was still there, but nothing like before, and there was relief from it for extended periods of time. The sad part about depression is when it lifts, you feel certain it's gone for good, only to have your hopes dashed a few hours later when it returns. I often think of depression as a major storm moving inland from the ocean. You can see it coming from the size and shapes of the clouds, but nothing prepares you for when it hits shore. Once the storm is gone, you are in the clear—not so with depression, the storm returns the next day, often stronger and more violent than before.

While I wasn't a fan of Rock & Roll Circus' manager Hugh Hardy, in some ways he helped me, especially in my early days in St Pat's. He called constantly to find out when I was getting out. He invested a small fortune in the band and after seeing them without their crazy guitar player, he finally realized that I was a key part of their sound. The staff told him I was making progress and only time would tell if and when I'd be well enough to return to the stage.

The band played a show in Dublin during my time in hospital. Some of the staff from my ward went to see them in a venue just a few miles away. The next morning around the nurses' station, I heard the girls talk about their big night out seeing this rock & roll band from Galway. Other than those who took my manager's calls, I'm not sure if the girls realized they were treating one of the band's members. At that point in time, I didn't exactly look like someone who, just a few weeks earlier, was prancing around a stage in a fancy sequined shirt launching a guitar into the air in front of a thousand people. To the nurses, I was just another young man desperately struggling to find the light in the darkness of depression.

A Couple of Angels

Two weeks into my treatment at St. Pat's, the staff nurse in charge said I had some visitors to see me in the café. I told her I wasn't expecting anyone, but she suggested I take a moment to greet them. I made my way to the café to find two girls who had come up from Galway to visit me. Mairead Foyle was one of the girls; I don't remember the name of the other. I knew Mairead pretty well as her brother was in my class at St. Enda's. The other girl I just knew from seeing her during my gigs around Galway.

The girls heard from a mutual friend that I was sick. They had summer jobs and took a day off from work to hitchhike the 120 miles from Galway on one of those miserable wet and cold Irish days where the rain fell horizontally.

The hospital was spotlessly clean, but it had that large institutional atmosphere with high ceilings and polished tiles smelling of disinfectant. The long corridors echoed with the voices of poor souls who were in various levels of distress. Most of the patients were older, and the ones who were not severely ill were allowed to walk freely in certain areas. That must have made the young girls uncomfortable. How could a twenty-year-old who seemed to have it all end up in such a sad place?

My heart filled with joy on seeing the girls and I couldn't believe they had come all that way just to see me. They talked about all that was going on in Galway: the dances, the bands that were playing in the various venues around town, the romances and breakups. It was a bit of normalcy in abnormal circumstances.

After an hour, I was exhausted, so the girls set off to make the long trip back to Galway in the still-pouring rain. It was an act of kindness I can never forget and better than any medicine. I did thank the girls months later when I was back in Galway but they will never fully understand how much they helped me. I'm not a very religious person, but I do believe Mairead and her friend represent what religion, spirituality and Christianity should be all about. I will always think of them as a couple of angels. Maybe there's a song waiting to be written about them! As I progressed in St. Pat's, other friends made the trip to Dublin to see me and lift my spirits.

A Weekend Pass

After two weeks at St. Pat's, I was allowed a weekend pass. It was a coveted document as it was the first indication you were on the way back to join the real world. Patients had to have an exit interview with Mr. Johnson, the head administrator of the hospital, before leaving the premises. He was an imposing man with a deep booming voice. He spent ages talking to me about avoiding the drink over the weekend. I began to wonder who was crazy. I had never taken a drink in my life and certainly had no intention of starting on my weekend pass. Did rest of the staff at St. Pat's also believe I was a recovering alcoholic? It was sad to see some of those standing in line having their weekend pass revoked before they left the hospital because Mr. Johnson felt they were not ready for the outside world. In just one second, their hopes were dashed.

My sister Ger, who lived and worked in Dublin, picked me up from the hospital and we went straight to the Dublin Zoo. It was a very strange day. Once the novelty of being out of St Pat's wore off, I began to experience terrible anxiety. I was safe behind the walls of St. Pat's but now I was in a world with no controls or boundaries. The chaotic traffic and the sights and sounds of the city streets sent my mind spinning uncontrollably.

I was happy when I got back to the hospital the following night. There were many like me, glad to walk back through the gates of St. Patrick's after their weekend pass. I was becoming institutionalized and I wasn't alone. My sister Ger is an amazing person. She kept a strong exterior during the weekend, but it was hard watching her young brother struggle trying to re-engage in the real world at the most basic level. She saw I had a hard time staying afloat and worried if the old Seamus would ever return.

A week later, I felt much better and went back home to Galway on an extended weekend pass. It was an up-and-down few days, much like my time with my sister Ger the previous week, with the anxiety coming and going.

The center of Galway is a small bustling place with just a few main streets. As I made my way through town, I ran into several friends who knew I was sick and they wished me well.

There was one particular character, Aggie Dowling, who crossed the street when he saw me. Aggie had long flowing fair hair and was as hip a character as you could meet. He had a swagger in his walk, like the Fonz in Happy Days, that made it clear he was the leader of the pack. He was also a real tough guy, feared by many, as it didn't take much to provoke him into a full-out brawl, especially after a few drinks. Despite his aggressive tendencies, Aggie loved the music and often came to see me perform. I didn't know what was going on when he walked up to me on the street. In his thickest Galway accent, he said, "Seamy, how is it fuckin' goin' like? I heard you were in St. Pat's." I told him I was dealing with a bad bout of depression but I expected to be back in action soon. His reply was classic Aggie: "Seamy, great to fucking see ya. Sure, there's nothing fucking wrong with ya. Take care, man." With that, he walked back to his buddies and continued up Shop Street with that distinctive swagger and his fair hair blowing in the Irish wind. I'm sure Aggie had no idea what the word depression meant, but he was relieved that his favorite long-haired fucking weirdo guitar player was on the mend. He saw the normal in me that I was having difficulty seeing.

After that weekend in Galway, I went back to the hospital and was about to be released permanently when I got chronic laryngitis. I couldn't move my head for two days. It was just about gone when it came back twice as bad as the first dose. When all was said and done, it extended my visit to St. Pat's to five weeks in total. The extra time in the hospital was probably a good thing. My medications were drastically reduced and I was able get ready for discharge under the close eye of my psychiatrist and the amazing staff at St. Pat's.

I got the best of care in the hospital. It was unusual for St. Pat's to have a patient so young suffering depression and anxiety. In a way, that's very sad, because I'm sure there were many young people like me around Ireland suffering in silence who would have benefitted from the treatment I received. Because of the stigma attached to mental illness, the inability of most people to recognize its signs and a lack of willingness to talk openly even when they did, many lives were needlessly lost. I was one of the lucky ones; I had a dad who saw past the stigma and wasn't afraid to talk openly about mental illness. Many weren't so lucky.

Going into a psychiatric hospital is a traumatic event, especially for a young person. You are mentally distressed and wonder if you will ever get better. The discharge from hospital came with its own challenges. In my case, after being in a safe and controlled environment for five weeks, I was terrified I wouldn't be able to adjust to the world outside the gates of St. Pat's.

When I arrived back to Galway, I was free of chronic depression, but it was a shaky balance at best. There were many times when I felt I was on the verge of slipping back into the darkness. I was afraid I'd let Dad and sisters down by doing so. That's the sad thing about depression—you see the world in such a distorted way and worry about the wrong things.

Rock & Roll Circus kept my place in the band open despite my two-month hiatus. They had various Galway musicians fill in for me. I met up with Ja and Liam to figure out a strategy for getting me back on the road. They handed me a huge wad of ten-pound notes paying me half salary for the time I was in hospital. I was completely taken by surprise as that was unheard of in the music business—it showed me they cared and they valued me as an integral part of the band.

By late 1974, the band was not traveling quite as much, and the big national push was coming to an agonizing end. As great as it is to be part of a band gaining momentum by the day, it's heartbreaking when you see the crowds diminish and the dream of success and stardom slip through your hands and vanish before your eyes. We started playing back around Galway more often which was good for me as the family could keep an eye on me. By early fall, Rock & Roll Circus had decided to call it quits, but we were to have one last fling and it would change my life forever.

The Audition

We got a call from our manager that Joe Doherty, a Mayo man living in America who owned a big club, was coming to audition us for a possible tour of America. He suggested we learn some country and western music as that's what Doherty was mainly looking for. We knew Rock & Roll Circus was coming to an end but a trip to America sounded like the perfect finale since American rock and roll was at the very core of the music we played. So it was off to the record shop to buy the country and western music we all hated so much. Irish country and western music was a horrible, diluted version of American country music. It was the music loved by many living in the rural parts of Ireland, and they constituted the vast majority of Irish immigrants to America. Within four days, we had a full set of songs including: "A Mother's Love's a Blessing," "Gentle Mother" and just about every song that mentioned the death or loss of a loved one.

We didn't know what to expect during the audition. Our manager Hardy was there with Joe Doherty, who turned out to be a tiny figure of a man dressed all in black with a white tie. His Mayo accent was overlaid with an American twang that included just about every cliché in the book. His slicked back, jet-black hair had an Elvis flare to it complete with carefully groomed sideburns. His larger-than-life persona was in such contrast to his tiny stature. We were amused and enthralled by him and completely taken by his positive energy, something that was rare during the deep recession Ireland was experiencing then. He liked what he heard and was particularly taken by Liam's Elvis and Roy Orbison impersonations and my unusual guitar playing. We were booked on the spot for a three-week tour scheduled for November of 1974—less than a month away.

Dad and my sisters were nervous about me going to the U.S. It had only been four months since I left the confines of St. Pat's, but we were all in agreement I had nothing to lose. It was either play it safe and stay in Galway or throw caution to the wind and try and move on with my life and career. Despite our ups and downs as a band, we all got along. It was a comfort to the girls and Dad knowing the guys would keep an eye on me.

America

Growing up, America seemed a wondrous place. It had me from the first grainy black and white images of Rin Tin Tin and The Adventures of Kit Carson on our tiny black-and-white TV in the early '60s. But what impressed me most about America was the sun shining all the time—at least in the movies. By contrast, Galway seemed to be in a perpetual state of cloudiness, although many of those clouds were in my mind's eye.

My mother was fascinated by space travel and Muhammad Ali, or Cassius Clay, as he was known in the early sixties. Mam never missed a space launch no matter what time of day or night and sitting around as a family listening to the countdowns are moments I treasure. Those space launches and the landing on the moon represented the can-do positive attitude of America and its people. I'm not sure what the fascination with Muhammad Ali was—maybe it was his optimism and his good looks, but it was shared by many people all over the world.

On November 5, 1974, we set out on our American adventure. A sax player, Garret O'Dowd, came along to "augment" the group at the last minute. He was a super-talented musician and very funny, so he fit right in with the Circus.

It was the first time to America for everyone in the band. There was an excitement in the air you could almost touch. The legendary Irish band, The Chieftains, sat in the row in front of me. The adventure of a lifetime for me was old hat to them. They were embarking on their annual North American tour so it was just another day for their great band, while my head was spinning in anticipation of what was ahead of us.

As the plane descended on our approach to Kennedy Airport in New York, I looked out the window and saw a sprawl of houses that stretched for miles. In the distance, I could see the sun reflecting on the massive skyscrapers of Manhattan. This was a dream coming true in front of my eyes. All the movies and TV shows I had watched over the years were flashing through my mind. I was excited and terrified at the same time. Would I be able to handle it all?

Before collecting our luggage, we had to go through immigration. At Shannon Airport in Ireland, our manager gave us one directive, "No matter what happens, don't tell the immigration officials in America you are working there. Just say you are on vacation. That's what your visitor visa says." With four guitars and a saxophone, it was a hard sell to say we were on vacation. It was incredibly intimidating talking to the immigration officers. They had guns strapped around their waists, they weren't friendly, they were huge and they talked in loud voices with a tone that exuded authority.

Everything was going fine until Liam was asked by one of the officers, "What's the purpose of your visit, sir?" He had been coached to simply say one word: "pleasure." This was 26 years prior to 9/11. The Irish were very welcome in America so things should have been relatively easy. But Liam said in his full-on Galway accent, "Ah, sure, we're just going to play a few gigs around New York." We were absolutely stunned and figured our grand adventure had come to a screeching halt before we set foot outside the airport. The immigration officer did everything he could to conceal his laughing; you could see he was thinking, "What in the name of God are you thinking, Paddy?" But instead, he pulled a business card out of his pocket and handed it to Liam. It had the names of multiple New York bars including: The John Barleycorn, Flanagan's, and The Abbey

Tavern. "I know the guys who run these places, give them a call and tell them Arnie sent you. They might be able to help you out. Welcome to America, boys."

We were met at Kennedy Airport by Joe Doherty and his partners, Aidan McCaffery and Martin Joyce. The airport was chaotic with people arriving from all parts of the world. The Cazabon family and the folks that worked in a Chinese restaurant in Galway were the only people I'd ever seen that looked different from me. At Kennedy, everybody looked different. We were the odd ones out. The multiple languages being spoken resonated through the air like a wild symphony with each language its own instrument. The sight of thousands of people of every color and creed, many dressed in their native garb, was a feast for the eyes. My brain was on overload, but this time, in the best possible sense.

Aidan was from Galway and Martin from Connemara. Andy and I referred to our host as the Cowboys, an endearing term we often used growing up to describe people who danced to their own drum. They took great care of us from the very start of our odyssey, but the next several weeks with them was a walk on the wild side unlike anything I ever experienced before or since.

The Cowboys had two cars to take the band and our equipment to our motel in the Bronx. One of the cars was a maroon-colored Chrysler and the other a massive Buick. We felt like rock stars.

After loading our luggage and equipment into the cars, our hosts drove like maniacs, literally rear-ending each other, as we exited the airport. A litany of profanity, all with that American twang superimposed on their Irish accents, was all we heard during the hour-long trip to the Bronx.

The Van Wyck Expressway was four times larger than any road we had travelled in Ireland. Thousands of cars, huge trucks, busses, and gigantic black and white limousines twice the size of normal cars did a chaotic dance on the expressway at incredible speeds. We made our way onto the Major Deegan Expressway in the South Bronx. On each side of the roadway, tall dark brown apartment blocks, each at least thirty or forty stories high, jutted into the air. The Cowboys told us this was a place to stay away from at all costs. Racial tensions were high in the early '70s and certain places were described as no-go areas by our hosts, especially for a few young lads just off the boat from Ireland.

We were booked into a small motel in the Bronx. It wasn't exactly the Ritz, but we didn't care—it was a place to lay our weary heads after the long journey. Once settled, we were taken to the Capital Diner on Kingsbridge Road for a meal. When I was in hospital in Dublin, I took a liking to liver, a strange choice of food for a finicky eater like myself. It must have been the meds I was taking. In Ireland, liver is normally served in small portions. At the Capital Diner, the waitress put almost an entire calf on my plate. It was absolutely delicious, but I could only eat one-third of it. Before leaving Ireland, a friend who had spent a summer in New York said, "Seamus, everything is just bigger in America." He wasn't kidding.

The next day, the Cowboys drove us to a music shop to get the amps and drums we needed for our show. There were more expletives as they drove through Fordham Road in the Bronx at breakneck speed like they owned the place.

The Circus Comes to Town

A few days after settling in, the Circus got on the subway and headed to Manhattan. The noise from the ancient all-gray metal subway cars and the steel wheels against the iron tracks was deafening. I thought my eardrums would burst. The subway cars were filthy and covered with multi-colored graffiti.

We had heard all the stories and warnings about the subway: don't look at or talk to anyone, keep your money hidden in an inside pocket, and always be on alert for someone trying to snatch your belongings. Within a minute of entering the subway car, Liam was fully engaged with multiple characters telling them, much to their amusement and our horror, he was out from Ireland on tour with the Irish band Rock & Roll Circus. He had just broken all the unwritten rules of New York subway etiquette. But Liam was color-blind. He treated everyone the same and was intrigued by how many different ethnic groups were on the same subway car. Wouldn't it be wonderful if we all saw the world through Liam's eyes?

We emerged from the Times Square subway station to a whole new world. The trip from Kennedy Airport to the Bronx didn't prepare us for what we saw. We couldn't stop looking up at the enormous glass and steel buildings, one taller than the next. It was just like the movies, except it was even more mind-blowing in person. The streets were teeming with people moving around like ants in an ant mound. The constant sound of sirens, as police and fire trucks sped through the crowded roadways, created an atmosphere of chaos and mayhem.

Times Square was lined with movie theatres showing the latest pornography movies, Deep Throat and The Devil in Miss Jones, complete with graphic posters outside the theatres. Massage parlors and porno peep shows were sandwiched between the theatres. In the middle of all this were small shops selling everything from machetes to the latest electronic gear. The air was heavy with the smell of roasted nuts and hotdogs from vendors lining the streets. A constant column of white steam rose from huge vents in the middle of the road. The city felt like it was ready to erupt at any moment like the Old Faithful geyser at Yellowstone National Park.

We stopped into Manny's Music store on 48th Street. It's where Jimi Hendrix and The Beatles bought their guitars ten years earlier. The walls were adorned with autographed photographs of Hendrix, The Beatles and every star you could name. I felt like I was walking on hallowed ground. In particular, I could feel the ghost of my all-time guitar hero Jimi Hendrix.

I had never seen so many guitars in one place and Manny's was just one of about 20 music stores on 48th street. An American musician I met in Galway told me to look up "Billy" at Manny's. Billy was a five-foot-two African American. He loved my Irish accent and the way I played Irish tunes on the electric guitar—thus began a twenty-year friendship. From that day on, I got the royal treatment when entering Manny's.

Over the years, I met many music legends on 48th Street, including Chet Atkins, Mark Knopfler, Slash and Jaco Pastorius. Sadly, all those places are closed now but I still feel the presence of those music stores, and my buddy Billy, when I walk along 48th Street.

We moved on from Manny's after a few hours to a bar around the corner on 7th Avenue for a drink. It was a smoky place with darkened windows and an abundance of neon lighting on every wall. Outside the bar, there was an intimidating bouncer in a tuxedo who must have weighted 350 pounds. That should have been a signal that something wasn't right. Within moments, exotic women appeared out of nowhere wearing almost nothing. It was early November, so I was surprised to see the girls dressed like they were at the beach. They sat next to each of us rubbing us up and down. I wasn't exactly a magnet for the ladies, so I was delighted with myself when a heavily perfumed lady showered affection on me. My twenty-year-old heartbeat quickened with each passing minute. My new friend Amanda said, "Hey sweety, will you buy me a drink?" I said, "Sure, why not," even though I was just drinking Coca Cola. I bought Amanda two drinks. My part of the tab came to forty dollars—more than what I was making in Ireland for a week's work. It was even more expensive for the drinkers in the band. We had experienced our first American scam. We all shared a great sense of humor, and once we realized what happened, we fell over laughing comparing the different girls that befriended us. Poor Liam was mortified and was once again convinced he had committed a mortal sin.

Show Time

After returning from our Manhattan adventure, we moved from our motel to an apartment on the famed "Decatur Ave" in the Kingsbridge section of the Bronx. It's where many of the Doo-Wop bands of the '50s got their start singing on street corners. By 1974, the entire area was run down with most buildings looking like they were barely habitable. The Cowboys rented a furnished apartment for us. It was in rough shape with cockroaches proudly parading around every room, but we didn't care. The first thing we noticed was a small black and white TV that had shows running all day long. That was enough to make our drummer Andy fall in love with America. Tom and Jerry and Micky Mouse at every hour of the day; life didn't get any better. He was obsessed with Disney. The bars being open till 4 am made Ja and our sax player Garret happy. Shops that sold every kind of gadget and the diners with huge food portions kept Liam in his element. I had my music stores in the Bronx and Manhattan where I quickly became a regular. We each had our own thing. What could go wrong?

After a few days of adjusting to life in America, it was time to hit the stage at the Wagon Wheel where we were scheduled for a three-week residency. It was one of a slew of large bars like Dirty Nelly's and the Jug of Punch catering to the Irish immigrants who came to the U.S. in the late '60s and early '70s. By 1974, immigration had slowed to a trickle, so most of the clientele at the Wagon Wheel had been there for several years and were well-adjusted to life in America.

We took to the stage in our fancy shiny brown band suits, complete with velvet collars and pockets my mother had sewn. The crowd was used to bands playing mainly country and western music from Ireland, so we were a novelty. They were shocked to hear Rock & Roll Circus do everything from Roy Orbison to Hawaii Five-O. We did the occasional country number to keep everyone happy. Some of the audience loved us and some didn't know what to make of this bunch of misfits playing rock and roll. The Wagon Wheel customers, even the ones who weren't big fans, and the staff were beyond generous and we didn't want for anything. They wouldn't let us put our hands in our pockets. It was their New York, and we were their guests.

As the days progressed, we were each adopted by different customers. I was cared for by a girl from Queens, Barbara Gallo, and her friends. I went to her house for dinner one Saturday evening. Barbara's family was everything I imagined an Italian family to be, based on the Mafia movies I watched before coming to America. The family could not have been more welcoming, but from the moment I walked in the door, they were yelling at each other, at least from my perspective. The house was next to the elevated subway line, so every time a train roared by, their voices rose to a crescendo, matching the noise of the train. This ebb and flow of the conversation continued throughout the meal that consisted of spaghetti and meatballs. I had never eaten either in my life.

I did my best to eat the spaghetti without drawing attention to myself. But little, if any, spaghetti made its way from the large plate to my mouth before falling off the fork. Mamma Gallo, who immediately recognized my struggle, stepped in and proceeded to show me how to wind the noodles around my fork. I turned every shade of red with embarrassment. Making things even more uncomfortable, Mamma Gallo also decided I might marry Barbara, whom I just considered a friend with benefits. I made my escape immediately after dinner as I had a show in the Bronx that evening. I remember stopping at the Capital Diner on Kingsbridge Road and having a huge feed of pancakes and chips and vowing to never return to the borough of Queens.

Thanksgiving Mayhem

Dad had two sisters living in America, Rita and Nora. They emigrated in their mid-twenties, a few years before the Great Depression of 1929. Both were in New York, Nora in Brooklyn, and Rita in the Bronx. I met them once before coming to America when they were on a rare visit back home to Ireland. They were incredibly kind and a lot of fun, so I looked forward to spending time with them. Both loved Mam and Dad.

It was late November when Rita and her husband, Barney, picked me up on a Thursday morning from our Decatur Avenue apartment for Thanksgiving dinner at Aunt Nora's in Brooklyn. It was eerily strange to see the entire city come to a virtual standstill in the middle of the week. It felt like a Christmas Day in Ireland because everyone was off work and there was a festive atmosphere everywhere with people wishing each other Happy Thanksgiving.

We picked up Barney's sister-in-law Marge along the way. I literally had a pain in my ear by the time we got to Brooklyn. Marge was loud and obnoxious. I couldn't believe how rude she was to Rita and Barney, dismissing anything they said—after all, they were from Ireland, so Marge figured they knew nothing.

Aunt Nora's beautiful brownstone house in the Prospect Park area of Brooklyn looked like something from Sesame Street. It had a brown brick exterior and what was called a stoop outside the front door with four or five steps leading down to the street. When the weather was nice, families congregated on the neighborhood stoops creating a wonderful sense of community.

We were met at the door by Nora, a small plump lady with a big heart and funny as hell. Her husband died in his mid-forties, so she raised her children, Jim and Mary, as a single mom.

Once inside the house, the smell of roasted turkey took me back to our family Christmas dinners in Galway, but the amount of food at Nora's house made it feel more like a medieval banquet.

If it was loud in the car on the way to Brooklyn, the volume increased dramatically with the cast of characters assembled in Nora's home. It made my Italian friends in Queens seem quiet by comparison. Jim Buckley, a distant relative, sat at the head of the table. Buckley was a huge, bellicose, obnoxious man. Nora's son, Jim Daly, was there with his wife, Barbara, and their two boys. Jim was also a very large man, carrying the characteristic Kelleher beer belly. Unlike Buckley, he was a gentle giant, but he was also loud and called things exactly as he saw them. He was devoid of any filters. His wife was a lovely woman with the best Brooklyn accent in the world and not afraid to voice her opinion on any topic.

Nora's daughter, Mary, and her husband, Raymond, rounded out the eclectic group around the dinner table. Over the course of five hours, I witnessed confrontations I was sure would result in a serious injury or worse to one or more of the dinner guests. Buckley, Marge, Barbara, Mary and Jim proceeded to drink bottle after bottle of wine like cans of soda.

I came from a very quiet household where it was rare for anyone to raise their voice, especially during dinner. Between Marge displaying her contempt for anyone from Ireland and Buckley showing total disregard for every woman at the table, I felt the need to increase the dosage of medication I was still taking for my depression and anxiety.

Looking back on that first Thanksgiving in America, I realize there was another aspect to the get-together, one I didn't understand until many years later. Aunt Nora, Rita and Barney played host to a cast of characters who might not have been welcome in another house in Brooklyn or indeed anywhere in New York. Rita and Nora knew Marge would insult them, that Buckley would be rude and degrade every woman present and Nora's daughter would have too much to drink, but they were accepting of it all. It was just who they were. It was a lesson in kindness, tolerance, empathy and compassion.

Thankfully, nobody died during that Thanksgiving dinner, but I was very happy to get back to my apartment in the Bronx to meet up with my buddies from the Circus. Suddenly, despite being such odd balls, my fellow band members seemed very normal.

Discovering New York

As the weeks rolled on, there was friction in the band over financial issues. We had heated arguments that put stress on everyone, especially Liam, who was a bit overwhelmed with New York in the first place. He never quite settled in like the rest of us. He was a homeboy and missed his wife and kids, and the American food, even in its abundance, was getting to him. While each of us in the band had our own clique and discovered our own version of New York, Liam couldn't find his place. The novelty of New York was quickly wearing off.

Out of the blue, Liam told Ja he was going home. We had several weeks to go on our contract, so things got very tense. But Liam was on the verge of a breakdown so the Cowboys, after much consultation with Ja, agreed to let him off the hook and go home. It was better to release Liam from the contract than deal with the consequences of him staying in the Bronx, where something could go terribly wrong. On a cold November evening, Liam made his way to Kennedy Airport where he boarded an Aer Lingus plane for home.

We managed to get by without our fearless leader. The tension quickly disappeared after we worked out the finances of the band. There was no way to replace Liam's God-given voice and his rock-solid guitar playing. We did our best to fill the gap and the Cowboys found a local New York band to help us out on weekends. I became good friends with their guitar player, Tommy Sullivan. He introduced me to another side of America. Most Irish immigrants who arrived in New York in the 1970s and '80s congregated around specific Irish neighborhoods such as Kingsbridge and Woodlawn in the Bronx and Woodside in Queens. Tommy and his family lived in Brooklyn and seemed to be part of the larger America, and that appealed to me. For example, conversations around the dinner didn't always center around the Irish bars and the Irish community. They discussed politics and daily life in America. I was enthralled by that.

We were due to finish our tour in early December '74, but our hosts asked us to stay on until early January. We all agreed, knowing it might be our only chance to experience America. We also knew we had no bookings in Ireland for January and February.

It was hard being away from my family that Christmas, especially since it was the first one since Mam passed. I missed my sisters, Dad and my friends, but I was blessed to have Aunt Rita and Nora.

Christmas dinner, this time at Aunt Rita's in the Bronx, had the same misfits as Thanksgiving just a month earlier, but for some reason, I wasn't too bothered by all the ruckus. I found the humor in Marge being Marge, in Buckley being an asshole, and all the idiosyncrasies of those gathered around the table. Even though I had been in America just two months, I was changing. I wasn't yelling at the table, but I wasn't the shrinking violet everyone had seen just a month earlier. I had my opinions and wasn't afraid to express them. At one point, I told Buckley he was full of shit. There was a collective gasp from everyone at the dinner table. Rita, Barney and Nora enjoyed the subtle change in my personality. Buckley, not so much.

I had mixed feelings about going back home when the time came in early January to wind down our residency at the Wagon Wheel. While I missed my family in Ireland, the trip to America had given my confidence a boost. People were paying attention to my guitar playing. I was beginning to open up and engage with audience members and friends. I also enjoyed the fact that I could be anonymous in America when I chose to be. I could disappear into the crowd and didn't have to explain anything to anyone. There was nothing to remind me of the darkness of St. Enda's or St. Pat's, and the horrible strife that was still part of everyday life in Ireland wasn't on the news every day. Best of all, on most days, I was free from the demons of depression.

Before leaving America for home, I did my belated Christmas shopping for the family on Fordham Road in the Bronx. It is an extraordinary place with people from every corner of the world crammed into an area of a few square blocks. I was looking at a small pocketknife for my brother-in-law in a store when the salesman, who heard my heavy Irish accent, suggested I follow him to a side room where he got deadly serious saying, "You're from Ireland right?" I said, "Yep." He continued, "I hear there's a war going on over there. Maybe you want something more special." He took out an oversized black key and opened a closet filled with an assortment of weapons that would be the envy of any terrorist group. There were daggers with golden handles, assault rifles, swords three feet long, and implements of war designed to damage the human form in ways too gruesome to contemplate. His weapon of choice for me was a machete in an ornate shiny gold holster with a blade at least thirty inches long. All I could think of was going through customs in Ireland and trying to explain the machete at a time when the troubles in the North were at their very worst. I politely declined the weapons dealer. His intentions were good, but the IRA didn't need any help from Seamus Kelleher.

As we said goodbye to New York and our kind and quirky hosts, Joe, Aidan and Martin, I knew America had entered my soul and my psyche. I found somewhere where I could be me, a place where I could get a fresh start. With the lights of New York City fading into the distance as the Aer Lingus 747 jumbo jet climbed into the air, I replayed in my mind all that had happened in just a few short months. It was truly a great adventure.

From Boy to Man

There was great excitement upon my return to Galway. We had a ritual as a family that involved a trip to the pub after someone had been away, where the whole family gathered to catch up on things. Since there was no social media then, the pub was the main form of communication. Often, after a few drinks and some storytelling, the guitar came come out and there was a singsong.

Dad was eager to hear all about America. He had a fascination with the place. He was delighted to hear that I spent so much time and got along so well with his sisters, Rita and Nora, whom he loved dearly. He was most happy to see I had come a long way since he had last seen me only ten weeks earlier. My growing self-confidence and general optimism were things he hadn't seen before. In just a few short months, I had gone from boy to man.

We did our final show as Rock & Roll Circus at Seapoint Ballroom in Salthill a month after our return from America. It was the annual Debutant's Ball where all the college students came together for a night of wild celebration. The show was great and we certainly went out on a high note. Stepping off stage after playing to a crowd of well over a thousand frenzied students, I was fully aware I was blessed to be part of such an amazing band at a young age. I also knew for sure that being a professional musician was what I was destined to do for the rest of my life. There was no going back to life on the factory floor in SPS.

I started playing fill-in shows with bands around town. I got frequent calls to play with a local showband Murphy and the Swallows. The band was well-established and performed throughout Ireland five or six nights a week. Most of their music was in the country and western vein which I wasn't fond of, but their musicianship was second to none, and they let me do several of my rock and roll songs during their show. After a while, they talked about the possibility of me joining the band fulltime for a sizable weekly salary. At twenty years of age, that was an appealing offer but deep down inside, I heard a voice telling me, "Don't do it."

It was time for a change. America had opened my eyes beyond the insular Ireland still under the chains of bondage of the Catholic Church. I felt more confident in myself and decided that my struggles with depression, my dark memories of St. Enda's and my teenage years didn't have to define who I was. I liked the idea of a fresh beginning, an opportunity to forge my identity anew.

Heart to Heart

My favorite time of day was from 11 pm to 3 am. It was my depression-and-anxiety-free zone. That's when I sat in the kitchen and practiced for hours, endlessly repeating riffs on the guitar trying to increase the speed at which I played. Dad came home from work at around 2 am. To help him sleep, he boiled the kettle for a hot whisky after a long day at work. That five minutes when the kettle boiled was always a great time for the two of us to chat.

"Dad, I think it's time for me to go back to America," I said. It had to be hard for him to hear those words. Three months before she died, Mam called me into her room and said, "Seamus, if anything ever happens to me, will you make sure to take care of Dad?" I was surprised by the conversation as she was in good health then and there was no indication something might be wrong. I protested, "Mam, nothing is going to happen you." But I knew she needed to hear it from me so I promised her I would always take care of Dad. So, it was with all kinds of mixed emotions that I told Dad my plan. One part of me felt I was betraying my promise to Mam, but I also knew what Dad wanted more than anything was for me to get on with my life.

When my father had something serious to say to me, he called me Jim (the English for Seamus). Without lifting his head, Dad said as he stared into the hot whisky glass with the steam rising into the air, "Sure, Jim, you're old enough to make up your own mind about something like this. You know more about the music business than anyone around here." I told him I felt bad about leaving, not even a year since Mam died. Once again, as he had done all my life, he showed his undying unselfishness and his full support saying, "Seamus, you have no obligations here. I'll be fine, you need to get on with your career. The girls will help out around the house." He went on, "You're good about the drink and the drugs so you'll be fine as long as you keep an eye on that." It was only eight months earlier that we had a much harder conversation as I was heading to the psychiatric hospital in Dublin. This talk could have been just as hard, but he made sure it was easy.

What was in Dad's head when he drove me to Shannon Airport two months after our conversation? He was probably happy knowing I was staying with his sister Rita in America until I got settled. Was he sad that he wouldn't see me daily, especially at 2 am when we had our chat as he was having the nightcap? Did he pray that the depression would give me a break long enough to pursue my dreams as a musician, and did he hope that someday I would go back and get a proper education?

Farewell

In addition to saying goodbye to my four sisters and Dad, I was leaving Mary, my first true love. We were together almost a year. She knew I was carrying too much baggage and it was time for me to try and start over. I didn't know how long I'd be in America. It was to be at least six months as that's how long the visa was for. She never made me feel guilty about leaving and that was a wonderful gift from her. She was super smart, a great worker and had lovely friends, so I knew she would find her own way. I treasure our first kiss, our first intimate touch and her kindness and support when Mam passed. I'll always remember those wonderful Sunday afternoon dates with Mary sitting on the back of my Honda 50 as we explored the beauty and richness of the Irish countryside.

Right up to the moment I got in the car with Dad to go to Shannon airport, I second guessed what I was doing. I was taking a big risk, but I knew not getting on that plane had its own risks. I had a lump in my throat when I looked back at Dad standing at the Aer Lingus gate with his arms folded and his distinctive brown corduroy Trilby hat. I prayed he would be okay.

This journey to America was different from my first trip with the Circus five months earlier. I was on my own this time around. America was in the midst of a bad recession. I sold my beloved Sunburst Fender Stratocaster to pay for the airfare. I worked so hard to raise the money to buy it, but I knew there was no other way to fund my trip. I could buy a cheap guitar in America to get me by until I got established.

Aunt Rita and her husband Barney met me at Kennedy Airport. Barney had a great old Buick similar to the one the Cowboys had on my first trip to America. The car had a collection of solidified flies on the dashboard like notches in an old tree trunk telling its age. But it was a metaphor for both Rita and Barney. It was what was under the hood that mattered.

The excitement I experienced a few months earlier when I arrived at Kennedy was replaced by trepidation. As I got into Barney's car, I felt like throwing up. The drive to the Bronx was one of the longest I've ever experienced. I missed Mary, my family and my friends. I looked at my watch and it said 10 pm. It was still on Irish time, five hours ahead of U.S. Eastern Time. I wondered if my friends were at our local pub, Mulholland's, where there was great music every night. Invariably, I was called on stage to do a blues number. I had the stark realization that might never happen again. I was overcome with melancholy.

Barney and Rita lived in the Westchester Square area of the Bronx. Their house was also a brownstone, not unlike Aunt Nora's in Brooklyn. The neighborhood was predominantly Italian, Jewish and Irish American. I didn't drive, so the subway, just a few hundred yards from the house, was my means of transport. After a few days settling in, it was time to hit the streets of New York in search of a job.

Things were easier on my first trip to America as I was waited on hand and foot and had a steady paycheck from performing at the Wagon Wheel. This time around, I was like any other immigrant. I had to forge my own path. I spent the days going to one bar after another looking for work as a bartender. Because of the dreadful recession, there was little work to be had not just in New York but throughout America. Car factories in Detroit were laying thousands of people off each month. Manufacturing ground to a halt. America was winding down its involvement in Vietnam. Soldiers were returning to the cities and they were looking for work. The country had a lot of healing to do socially and economically.

The Longest Days

"Missing My Hometown," by Seamus Kelleher

My story starts back in '68 when my friends and I were young
Where we played guitars in the local bars not for pay but just for fun
I thought some day I'd make it big and I'd leave that little town
But I never though what it would be like if my friends were not around
I'm missing my hometown my friends, I'm missing my hometown
It's where I was born it's where I'm bound, I'm missing my hometown

The days were excruciatingly long. Every minute felt like an hour. During those first few months, I found myself constantly looking at my watch wondering what my friends and family were doing back in Galway.

Calling home was not an option as the cost of an international call was astronomical. After a week, I received a letter from home. I was excited to see my sister Maura's beautiful cursive writing on the blue airmail envelope. It was the first of many epistles from her, several of which I still have tucked away. Her letters were full of information about what was going on in Galway. She knew exactly what I wanted to hear about. I also received letters from several close friends including Brendan Glynn and my girlfriend Mary. I read each letter many times over.

After a month with no prospects of a job, I thought I had made a dreadful mistake by coming to America. The little savings I had were depleted and I was increasingly anxious. Then one weekend, I got a call from a musician I met during Rock & Roll Circus' time at the Wagon Wheel. He had a gig for me backing up his wife, Maureen, who was a "singer." The gig paid fifty dollars, enough to fund my job search for another few weeks. Barney drove me to the gig, which was at a Chinese restaurant on Fordham Road in the heart of the Bronx. I hated Chinese food and the smell of it made me sick to my stomach. It was an ominous start to the evening.

I set up my amplifier and tuned my guitar. Maureen arrived with her entourage minutes before we were to go on stage. She was probably in her late thirties but it was hard to know as there was a lot of makeup involved highlighting the contours of her face. She had a huge mane of blonde hair perked up with massive doses of Aqua Net super-hold hairspray. She was an Irish Dolly Parton, at least from a distance. Her husband went off to do his own gig close by and left me to accompany Maureen for what was without doubt the longest night of my musical career.

There was no rehearsal. It was straight into "A Pretty Little Girl from Omagh." She made Yoko Ono sound like Barbra Streisand. I honestly didn't think someone could sing so out of tune and not know it. I have a very good ear for music and never had difficulty backing somebody up, but I couldn't find too many notes on the guitar to match what was coming out of her mouth. I wanted the ground to swallow me up. I tried to sing a few songs myself, but all I knew was rock and roll, and the few people there did not want to hear that. We played for over four hours with two twenty-minute breaks. Maureen and her husband could not have been kinder to me, and in fairness, maybe I was just not the right person to accompany her. I got in a taxi to take me home at around three in the morning, just glad I had survived the gig. It was a hard-earned fifty dollars that bough me some extra time in America

After six weeks, I was desperate and running out of options. I dreaded the thought of leaving America with nothing to show for all my efforts. My mood was changing and I could feel myself slipping back into the darkness. I spent each day going into bars, coffee shops and restaurants desperate to find any kind of work. With each rejection, I felt an anxiousness that reached deep down into the pit of my stomach.

A Lifeline

Just when all seemed lost, I got a call out of the blue from Mike Colbert, a drummer from Galway. He had been living in the U.S. for many years making a decent living as a professional musician. "Mouse," as he was known, was five-foot tall, very fond of the drink and God knows what else. He had a wonderful personality that attracted people of all ages. He was especially popular with the women who hung onto every word that came out of his mouth like he was some kind of shaman. He was a hard worker and did six five-hour shows a week. Mouse partnered with another Irishman, Joe Buckley, and bought a bar in Rockville Center on Long Island. They called it the Jolly Tinker after a well-known song from the Clancy Brothers and Tommy Makem.

Mouse knew I tended bar in Galway before coming to America and asked if I would be interested in being their day bartender. I felt an instant sense of relief and the deep anxiety I felt began to lift right away. Rita and Barney were just as excited as I was. They worried about me as they could see my mood deteriorating with the rejection I experienced each day of the job search. To make things even better, Mouse recruited Ja Reedy, the bass player from Rock & Roll Circus, to come out from Ireland to join the band at the Jolly Tinker. Christy O'Connor, a great entertainer also from Galway who already lived in New York, was chosen to lead the band at the Tinker. Now, in addition to finding a job paying good money, I'd be surrounded by friends and familiar faces from my hometown. They were several years older than me but it was such a blessing to have them nearby.

Within a week of the phone call from Mouse, I started work at the Jolly Tinker in Long Island. Rockville Center is a long way from the

Bronx, so I rented a small room in a private house down the street from the bar. The rent was twenty-five dollars a week and it was nice and clean. Shortly after starting work at the Tinker, I got a call from a musician friend Sean Fleming saying I should get in touch with his buddy Steve who was starting a band. I met with Steve Lastra, a bass player, and his friend Glenn Dawn, a drummer, and we hit it off immediately. They were forming a three-piece band called Three of a Kind and wanted me to be their guitar player.

In the space of a few weeks, I went from being completely broke and playing in a Chinese Restaurant on Fordham to playing with a decent American band and working five or six days a week as the day bartender in the Jolly Tinker. And I was making a lot of money—more than I had ever made in my life. And best of all, I was busy and didn't have time to think about how much I was missing my family and friends in Ireland.

Sex on the Beach

Being a bartender in America was very different from Ireland. It wasn't just that the cocktail drinks were foreign to me, the people were different. In Ireland, my job was to pull a good pint of Guinness or make the perfect Irish coffee and that was it. I had to be nice to people, but it wasn't my job to entertain them. In America, I had to fully engage with every customer who came through the door. I was their sounding board on every subject, from infidelity and alcoholism to the latest TV shows and all things political. They loved my heavy Irish accent and wanted to hear my story; where I came from, my family, my hometown and why I came to America. Initially, this drove me crazy, but after a while, I took a liking to the storytelling and started adding bits here and there to make it more interesting. The better the story, the bigger the tips.

The customers were amused by how clueless I was when it came to mixed drinks. Screwdrivers, Godmothers, Godfathers, Whisky Sours and Sex on the Beach were just a few of the drinks I had to make. The ladies enjoyed seeing me blush with their "Sex on the Beach" cocktail requests. I think they ordered the drink just to see me squirm. I bought a little bartending book to help me along, but it was the customers who helped me develop my cocktail-making skills.

The Jolly Tinker was home to a host of colorful characters like Bob, an air traffic controller at Kennedy Airport. When he was off the clock, it was one long bender until he had to be back in action. He was an unbelievably smart individual and a wonderful storyteller with a great love and knowledge of American history. I learned so much about America on those long afternoons at the Tinker when it was just the two of us, as he anesthetized himself from the pressures of his job. He also had a room in the boarding house where I lived, so many days after work I walked him back to the house in his drunken stupor. He was never nasty, but like many alcoholics I had come to know during my bartending days in Ireland, he was just trying to dull his pain with the drink.

Bob was in the Tinker the day Eastern Airlines Flight 66 from New Orleans to Kennedy Airport crashed on approach killing 113 of the 124 passengers onboard. The bar was 15 minutes away from the scene of the tragic accident. I could see the sadness and utter devastation in Bob's eyes as the TV news flashed images of grieving families waiting at the airline arrival terminal for news of their loved ones. He knew he had to go into work the following day and deal with the tragedy and the heartache of his colleagues, while having the daunting responsibility of directing planes in one of the busiest airports in the world. My heart went out to the poor man.

There was another character who came into the bar a few days a week. He was not the full penny, but we put up with him since he didn't bother anyone. One Monday morning, he put a quarter in the jukebox to hear Olivia Newton-John but her beautiful music didn't come on. Jokingly I said, "Give it a kick, Steve." Now Steve was about three hundred pounds. He stood back as if he were about to kick a penalty at a football game and put his foot through the jukebox, demolishing it and sending colorful pieces of glass from one end of the bar to the other. There were bits of 45s strewn across the floor. I was stunned but in a calm voice said, "Steve, I think you better leave now before the owners come in and I would advise you to avoid this place for a few months." That was the last I saw of him. Despite their anger on hearing about the jukebox, the owners took pity on Steve and never bothered to press charges.

The staff at the Jolly Tinker were great. They treated me like a "Greenhorn," a term used to describe someone just off the boat or plane from Ireland. After a few months, when I settled down and got to know everyone, the waitresses were teasing me one Saturday night after work and asked if I had ever "done the business." I was honest and told them no as my face turned a bright red. A few days later, Tina, one of the waitresses, took me back to my room. She was on a mission of mercy. Tina accomplished her task and we never went out again after that. It was something she had to do, and it was done. There were no bad feelings or emotions involved. It wasn't exactly the way I wanted my first intimate experience to go, but I survived the ordeal and was thankful that part of the education of Seamus was complete.

My band Three of a Kind got very busy. We went from playing a few gigs a month to performing five nights a week all over Long Island and New York. When we played in the Bronx, I stayed with Rita and Barney. They kept my room open for me.

I went to the post office every month and sent a postal money order to Dad for a few hundred dollars. As tough as things were in America, they were worse in Ireland. Dad sent several letters thanking me for my contributions. It felt good to help out and I was honoring my pledge to Mam to take care of him.

I made good money bartending and playing in the band and still didn't drink or smoke. Other than the one-night fling with Tina, romance was nonexistent, so my living costs were minimal. The bartending job came to an end after several months. As the recession continued to take its toll, the owners of the Jolly Tinker wanted to try out an extremely well-endowed blond bartender, hoping to attract the younger male clientele. The timing was good as I was exhausted working five nights at the music and five to six days bartending. I often got home at 4 am from gigs only to get up a few hours later to bartend. After the job ended, I still spent a lot of time in the Tinker as I remained great friends with the band and the owners. They insisted that I go into the kitchen to make meals for myself. I was incredibly grateful for the start they gave me in America.

A Letter from Dad

I got a letter from Dad in September 1975 telling me to stay in America if I could as there was nothing in Ireland for me. He listed all the factories that closed, resulting in high unemployment all over Ireland and particularly in Galway. He also said one of my musician friends was a passenger in his taxi and said how hard it was to get work and the pay was dismal. After much deliberation, I decided to stay in America, at least till things turned around in Ireland. As long as I kept a low profile, the chances were the immigration authorities would leave me alone.

My relationship with Mary had already begun to fade and the realization that I would be staying in America longer than originally planned was the final straw. There had been no set time for me to return to Ireland when I left Galway, but a long-distance relationship at that time was difficult as you didn't have the communications options we have these days with the internet and social media. Mary was my first love and set the bar high for whatever was to follow. She was a shining light at a time when I was consumed with darkness. There was no official breakup; we both just moved on.

After six months in America while still living on Long Island, I decided it was time to study music more seriously. It was one of the reasons I left Ireland in the first place. I enrolled at the American Institute of Guitar in Manhattan, next to Carnegie Hall. After studying classical guitar for several months, I studied at the Mannes Conservatory of Music, located in a beautiful old mansion on the upper East Side. I was intimidated when I first went there as the school was for the elite musicians in New York and I was not one of them—at least not yet. I studied music theory one-on-one with Leo Edwards, a wonderful African American gentleman. He was a dapper dresser and always had a perfectly ironed shirt, a spiffy jacket and a colorful bow tie to match. He was very patient with me and saw past some of the basic music fundamentals I was missing.

Mr. Edwards set me up with a piano teacher Mrs. Powers, considered one of the best teachers in New York. During some of our lessons, she put a white sheet over my hands and the keys of the piano so I couldn't see what I was doing. She wanted me to feel the instrument. Like Mr. Edwards, she was patient and supportive. My goal at the Mannes Conservatory was to get to the point where I could enroll fulltime in music college. I knew it would take a few years to get there but I had a plan. The tuition was high at the conservatory and there were no scholarships available to me, but I was making good money and figured I was investing in my future.

I stayed on Long Island for close to a year after the bartending job ended, but most of my band's work shifted to the Bronx, Brooklyn and Queens. I also had a long commute from Long Island for my music classes in Manhattan. Rita and Barney suggested I move back in with them for a while. They missed having me around and I was happy to come back to their lovely home and their wonderful company. They set up their basement as a lovely little apartment where I had my privacy.

To say Rita and Barney spoiled me was an understatement. Rita had my clothes washed and ironed each day and Barney drove me anywhere I needed to go. I think they enjoyed having a young person around as their three children were living out West. I became their fourth child. The three of us spent many hours sitting on their back porch teasing each other about where we were from in Ireland and talking about life in general. I especially loved hearing stories from Rita about what it was like growing up in rural county Kerry with her siblings including my dad.

I don't know what I would have done without Rita and Barney. I still had many days when the depression was lurking below the surface. They knew what I went through before coming to America. They gave me all the space in the world to do my own thing but there was great comfort for me and also for Dad and my sisters, knowing they were close at hand.

A Difficult Day

The one thing holding me back from executing any long-term plans was my visa status. My visitor visa expired after six months in America. The intent was to use some contacts I had been given prior to leaving Ireland to help secure legal status in the form of a Green Card. From my time bartending and the solid income from music, I quickly put aside money to start the legal process. I paid over two thousand dollars, a lot of money then, to a well-known New York immigration attorney. I was promised I wouldn't have too much difficulty securing the Green Card that would eventually allow me to become a citizen. Despite my attorney's optimism and willingness to take my money, my application was denied. It was devastating news as I was in America well over a year by then and felt like I was making progress on all fronts. I was utterly deflated when I walked out of the lawyer's ornate office in midtown Manhattan.

I knew without a visa I could not go home and expect to get back into the U.S. I missed my family and friends terribly and had a growing fear that something might happen to my dad before I had an opportunity to see him again.

Shortly after my visa application was denied, two of my sisters made it out to New York for a short visit. It was great spending time with them in the city I had come to love. I took pride in showing them around and introducing them to the people who were now part of my American family. But it was incredibly hard seeing them get back on the plane not knowing when or if I would be able to go back to Ireland. I had the money in my pocket to pay for a return airline ticket, but without a visa, it was going to be a one-way trip if I got on that Aer Lingus plane with my sisters.

License to Roam

My friend Steve from Three of a Kind grew tired of driving from Long Island to the Bronx to pick me up for shows. When I turned 21, he suggested I learn to drive.

Other than my Honda 50 scooter, I had never driven a motorized vehicle. Once I got my provisional license, Steve gave me several hair-raising lessons in his enormous Buick under the elevated subway lines in the Bronx. Barney also took me out on the road many times. After multiple lessons I took my driving test and passed. Getting a driving license was of huge importance as it provided me with a form of ID. Without a Green Card, I feared if I was stopped by the police for any reason, I could be reported to the immigration authorities. Having a driver's license made it less likely they would question my legal status.

I found a car advertised on Long Island. It was a big white Plymouth Duster with twenty thousand miles on the odometer and not so much as scratch on it. To me it was a brand-new rocket ship. I paid twenty-eight hundred dollars cash for the car. I don't remember driving home from the dealership. It was the first time I had driven alone. I was terrified, but it was a pretty straight shot highway-wise and I made it back to the Bronx alive.

Two days later, I got a call from Steve saying we had a last-minute booking at Rosie O'Grady's in the Wall Street area of Manhattan. He didn't have time to pick me up. That meant driving into Manhattan on my own during rush hour traffic on a Friday evening. The GPS hadn't been invented, so I did my best to follow the detailed hand-written directions Barney gave me. But with all the highways converging I found it incredibly confusing to the point of panicking. Cars whizzed by on every side honking their horns, giving me the finger, and opening their windows to call me an asshole and a mother f---ker in response to my erratic driving. I must have lost ten pounds during the trip, but eventually I made it to Rosie O'Grady's in one piece, at least physically. Steve was waiting for me and was delighted I had completed my first real driving test. While it got him off the hook in terms of driving me places, he was happy I now had freedom to experience America on my own terms.

Having a car was an instant game changer. It allowed me to branch out beyond my immediate surroundings in the Bronx. I didn't have to ride the subways at all hours of the night with a guitar in hand risking life and limb. The car also allowed me to hear bands performing all over the city and, most important of all, to meet others involved in the music business. It drastically accelerated my assimilation into the music business and the American way of life. Word travelled fast that I had a set of wheels, and since I didn't drink, I quickly became the much-in-demand designated driver for my friends who were fond of the beer.

After two years in America, I decided to get my own apartment. I knew Rita and Barney's children wanted them to move out West and I was afraid I was holding them back. I rented a sub-basement apartment in the Riverdale section of the Bronx, a nice area with beautiful tree-lined streets. I found it hard leaving Rita and Barney. They had been so good to me, and we had shared so many great times. But I knew it was time and the right thing to do.

A year after I moved out, Rita and Barney finally made their move to California. I was sad to see them go but relieved and happy they were reconnecting with their kids while they still had their health. It was hard for Rita's sister, Nora, as they were incredibly close: soul mates as well as sisters. I promised Rita and Barney I would pop out to Brooklyn to see Nora from time to time, something I did until the day she left Brooklyn in the early 1990s to live with her son in upstate New York.

Romance

There were several short-lived romances during those early years in America. When I was living with Rita and Barney, I got a lot of teasing from them whenever a new lady entered the picture. There were no cell phones then, so they were responsible for taking phone messages for me. I had different scripts for them to read depending on if the caller was Deirdre, Shannon or Barbara. The most notable romance was with Trish, a lovely girl from Philadelphia. I met her during my tenure at the Jolly Tinker where her uncle did a lot of the carpentry work. We were just good friends for a few years but then sparks began to fly, and I fell head over heels. She was beautiful and incredibly funny.

Trish came to visit me several times when I moved into my apartment in the Bronx. We shared many happy days enjoying some of the craziness and excitement that only a city like New York can provide. One weekend evening sitting at the sidewalk section of Friday's, a restaurant on First Avenue, a taxi came flying up on the sidewalk just a few yards from us. Mercifully, nobody was hurt, but all kinds of yelling went on between the taxi driver and the pedestrians who came close to meeting their Maker that day. Within a few minutes of the near catastrophe, people were back to their burgers and fries like nothing had happened. Trish and I found the whole thing incredibly amusing. Long-distance relationships are hard to maintain though, and since she lived in Philadelphia, after a while it fizzled out.

Heroes

When living in the Bronx, I took full advantage of the opportunity to see some of the biggest names in music. I was a regular at Madison Square Garden where I saw Eric Clapton, Led Zeppelin, Queen, Thin Lizzy, Aerosmith, Jethro Tull, Rush and Rory Gallagher. It was like going to school each night when the lights went down at the Garden to the roars of twenty thousand music fans as our heroes took the stage. The air was thick with the aroma of marijuana. "High" times indeed.

On a beautiful summer's night, I went to see one of my favorite guitarists and biggest influences, the great B.B. King, who was performing at one of the Schaefer Beer concerts in Central Park. I walked into the venue early and saw some open seats at the very front. So, in all my innocence, I sat down right in front of the stage. I was surprised that nobody had taken advantage of the amazing seats up front. There had to be five thousand people or more at the concert. As darkness descended, the remaining seats did fill up.

B.B. King and his band took the stage and instantly the crowd was on their feet. Half an hour into his set, B.B. said, "I want to thank you all for being here with me tonight, and in particular, my family seated right in front of me." It suddenly hit me; I was the only white person in the front row. I'm sure the family wondered who this young kid with a red face and freckles was, and what the hell was he doing sitting in the section reserved for B.B. King's family? But I was welcomed with open arms and had one of the very best nights of my life watching the master of the blues at work.

An Act of Kindness

After four years in America, my hands continued to be tied because of my lack of legal status. I was still playing music with Steve. With the addition of a new drummer, we changed the name of the band from Three of a Kind to American Way, but musically I was ready for something different. I took a leap of faith and left the band in 1979.

Within a short while, I was approached by my good friend, Sean Fleming, to record an album. Sean and his bass player, Chris Ebneth, were well known and highly respected in New York's music scene. They worked as a duo at Flanagan's Irish Bar on 66th Street and First Avenue in Manhattan. The energy in their performances was out of this world—they sounded like a six-piece band. I was thrilled to be asked to record with them. In addition to me, there was Paddy Higgins, a great drummer from Galway, Skip Krevens, a crazy-talented pedal steel player and a lovely keyboard player, Dave Prouty. The album was called Tripping the Dew.

Around the same time, I applied to a music degree program at Montclair State College in New Jersey. I had to do auditions on classical guitar and on piano in addition to math and English exams. That proved difficult as I had been out of school for seven years. When I received the letter from the admissions office at Montclair State College, I jumped for joy when I read the words, "Congratulations Seamus Kelleher, you have been accepted into the undergraduate program in Music Therapy at Montclair State College." Along with fulfilling a dream, going to college fulltime opened up the possibility of getting a student visa.

But then I ran into a major snag. The immigration authorities would not change my status given that I spent four years in the U.S. as an illegal alien. I went to the immigration office in New York in person to plead my case but to no avail. Not only that, a few weeks after my visit to their offices, I received a notice in the mail saying I had a month to leave the county voluntarily or I would face deportation. That letter was a bullet to my heart. I literally couldn't breathe and was utterly devastated. I didn't know where to turn and stared at that letter for over an hour, reading it several times over.

As luck would have it, a few days later, I ran into a lovely couple in New York at one of my shows. They knew me from seeing me perform around the city. I told them about being accepted to college but said it wouldn't happen now because of my visa situation. The girl said her sister worked at the U.S. Embassy in Dublin and maybe there was a way to solve my dilemma. The next day, she called her sister, who said if I went back to Dublin right away and met with her, things would work out. My friend couldn't give me any more information than that. I had nothing to lose at that point. I couldn't continue life as an illegal alien, looking over my shoulder all the time, now that the immigration authorities knew where I lived. I was about to take a huge risk.

Home at Last

In mid-December, I booked a ticket home and was on my way to Kennedy Airport. I was about to see Dad and the girls after almost five years and I'd be home for Christmas with the family. I could barely contain my excitement as I got on the plane, but deep down I feared that if things didn't work out at the embassy, I wouldn't be able to come back to America. I was filled with a strange mix of excitement and deep apprehension.

I arrived in Dublin Airport on a cold and frosty December day. My sisters Toni and Carol picked me up. I wasn't the biggest hugger, but both girls got a massive hug from their only brother. But we had no time to get lost in the emotions of the moment. We drove straight to the American Embassy to meet my contact about the visa. I was painfully aware this one meeting could change everything.

My heart rate quickened as I walked through the elaborate white marble facade of the Embassy with its huge American Flag blowing in the blustery Irish weather. There was a giant photo of President Jimmy Carter on the lobby wall. I was ushered into a small office to meet with the woman whose sister I met in the New York bar a few weeks earlier. I literally spent ten minutes at the Embassy and walked out with my student visa. When I got back into the car, I stared at the visa in disbelief. An act of kindness by someone I didn't even know had just changed the trajectory of my life.

It took a while for it all to sink in. I could breathe freely for the first time in years. No more worries about someone reporting me to the immigration authorities, no more looking around the corner as the number of raids on Irish bars escalated. If I needed to go back to Ireland for any reason, I could buy a ticket and be on Irish soil in a little under six hours and be able to return to America when I wanted.

The drive from the American Embassy to Galway with Toni and Carol was the strangest trip I have ever taken. Part of me was on cloud nine because of what had transpired at the Embassy and the excitement of seeing my sisters who I love so dearly after so long. But I felt like a stranger in my own land. The landscape was unlike anything I had seen in almost five years. The palate of green fields on either side of the road jumped out at me like the colors in a Van Gogh painting. I'd forgotten what Ireland looked like. It was like I was seeing everything for the first time.

For the better part of my first year in America, all I could think of was my friends and family in Galway. But at some point, I knew I couldn't live in two places at once. I forced myself to focus exclusively on my life in America. Unlike most Irish immigrants in the U.S., I had little interaction with Irish people in my day-to-day life. I lived far away from New York's Irish neighborhoods and ninety percent of my shows were in American bars. Essentially, I blocked out any connection to the Ireland I grew up in. I had left the trauma of my teenage years far behind.

Upon our arrival in Galway, I walked into the house I left years earlier and felt a rush of emotions. I was half expecting to see my mother standing in the kitchen. When Dad walked in the door after a taxi run, he simply said "how're ya." We didn't hug or shake hands—that's not what an Irish father and son did, but I was just about able to hold back the tears. I was so relieved to see him looking well and happy. The moment I dreamt about for years had arrived. I worried so much that I might never see him again. Judging from his face, Dad was the happiest man in the world at that moment. The girls were teasing me about my "American" accent, but Dad said, "For feck's sake, will ya stop, it's the first time I can understand a word he's saying." Before leaving Ireland, I didn't talk much and when I did, I muttered a lot in half-baked sentences. What little self-confidence I had was beaten out of me by the miserable bastards at St. Enda's. That lack of self-confidence didn't fly in New York. Rita and Barney and my friend Steve from Three of a Kind insisted that I learn to speak up and engage fully in conversation. Dad and my sisters clearly approved of the more outgoing Seamus.

During my two-week stay, I met up with all my old friends, many of whom had also left Ireland during the mid '70s to work in England and were home for the holidays.

Spending Christmas with the family after being away for almost five years was special. Much of the attention during those Christmas gatherings was focused on me. Dad and the girls were delighted to see me in good mental and physical health. The last time they had seen me, I was getting on a plane to go to America and nobody, including myself, knew if I had sufficiently recovered from my nervous breakdown and the trauma of my Mam's passing to take on such an adventure.

Return to Darkness

I arrived back in America early January full of energy and ready to take on the world. My plan was to continue my music studies in preparation for college the following September. I had no problem going through immigration with my new student visa. It was a great feeling when the immigration officer said, "Welcome back, sir, and good luck with your studies."

But after a few days, I knew something wasn't right. The depression was back with a vengeance, and it was bad. I was devastated as I had been relatively free of the darkness for close to three years. Aunt Nora insisted I stay with her for a few days in the hope I would snap out of it. She took great care of me but grew increasingly concerned as I became more depressed and agitated—a lethal combination. Nora could see I needed professional help and suggested I go back to Ireland for a while to be with the family. Just like my Dad five years earlier, she recognized I was in crisis.

Nora got special sleeping medication for me from her doctor before putting me on the plane home. I slept through the entire flight. Before we landed in Shannon, I was awakened by the stewardess who informed me that it was the worst transatlantic flight she had been on in her thirty-year career. The turbulence were so awful throughout the six-hour flight that no food or drink was served and no trips to the bathroom permitted.

I was met by Dad at the arrivals terminal in Shannon. My triumphant return to Ireland just a few weeks earlier was short-lived. After impressing my friends and family with my success in America, I was back in Galway in the deep fog of depression. I knew Dad was worried, so I pretended I just needed to rest up for a while. But he could see through my bravado and read the signs of depression better than me. He was worried sick.

It was determined by the family I'd stay with my sister Geraldine as she was at home minding her two little girls. The depression was intense even when I went back on the medication under the direction of our local doctor, Greg Little. It can take several weeks for antidepressants to kick in. It's a vulnerable time for anyone who is struggling with depression. As is often the case with people who reach that point, I felt I was a burden to everyone, and I had no reason to live. I was full of sadness and self-loathing. The beauty of Ireland that had brought me such joy a few weeks earlier faded into complete darkness. The Van Gogh like palate of greens that I marveled at seemed grey and black. I just wanted the pain to end. There were many days I wished I was dead.

It's hard to define what depression feels like but author William Styron in his book Darkness Visible: A Memoir of Madness, said, "The pain of severe depression is quite unimaginable to those who have not suffered it, and it kills in many instances because its anguish can no longer be borne. The prevention of many suicides will continue to be hindered until there is a general awareness of the nature of this pain."

My mental pain and anguish continued unabated for days on end. One evening, my sisters, their significant others, and Dad gathered for a family dinner in an effort to cheer me up. It was hard to get everyone together as they all had busy lives, so these family gatherings were traditionally festive and a fun time. There was the usual banter across the table with a lot of laughter and teasing, along with discussions on politics and the news of the day. During dinner, I had the sensation of floating over the table looking down and wondering why I couldn't be "like them." I did my best to hold in the tears during dinner, but after a while, I started sobbing uncontrollably. The hardest part was Dad seeing me in such a bad way. That evening, I didn't want to go on living like that. I couldn't bear Styron's "anguish" any longer.

Gradually I began to improve. Each day was a little brighter. I received a letter from Chris Ebneth, Sean Fleming's bass player, saying that Sean had been invited to tour Ireland that summer and they wanted me to be part of the band. The news lifted my spirits although I knew I still had a long road ahead of me before taking the stage.

Taking Control

I went back to the Greg Little after three weeks in Galway. In addition to being a wonderful doctor, he was a family friend and knew me well from the music. In his usual pragmatic way, he said, "Seamus, you left Ireland five years ago to go to America. You came home and saw things had changed. Your dad and sisters moved on with their lives after your mam's death, but in many ways, you haven't. Things are frozen in time for you, at least on the Irish side of the equation." He said it was natural to be going through the emotions I was feeling but what he said next rattled me, "Seamus, it's time to grab the bull by the horns and get back on that plane now or I'm afraid you never will." I was tempted to get all defensive, but I knew Greg was speaking the truth. I went straight from his office to the travel agent and booked a ticket back to America. Within a week, I was on my way to New York terrified that this would be an endless cycle continuing throughout my life. Was my life going to be like Mr. Duigan's at St. Pat's with recurrent bouts of depression and darkness landing me back into hospital every few years?

From Kennedy Airport, I got a bus to my apartment in the Bronx. I knew the first few days would be make or break time. The temptation was to leave the television on all day to keep my mind occupied, but I knew that I had to fight this thing head on or, as Greg said, "grab the bull by the horns." I wrote down a daily routine that included getting up at 9 am, having a boiled egg and toast for breakfast, followed by a half-an-hour exercise, a walk outside, and then a few hours of practice on guitar. I allowed myself two hours of TV each day. I knew I had to stay away from the bed. Oversleeping made my depression worse.

I talked to the doctor about medications before leaving Ireland and we agreed I would cut down the antidepressants to a minimal dose after a few weeks as long as I was feeling okay. Only then could I consider getting in a car and going back to work

Those first few weeks back in America were difficult, but I began to see positive signs of recovery and I was able to reduce the medication. The hardest part of the ordeal was getting out of bed in the morning not knowing what the day would bring. Most evenings I was free from depression. After a month, I felt I had taken back control of my life. I was back driving and well enough to do gigs with various singers and bands in the New York area.

Given my bout with depression, I wasn't sure what to do about school. The student visa would only remain valid if I started college within a year. All I could do was take it one day at a time. I wasn't quite ready to start college yet.

What helped lift my spirits most was the impending tour of Ireland with Sean Fleming scheduled from June through August of 1979. Sean was using mostly the same band that was on the album we made a few months earlier. I was over the moon. This was an opportunity to play with these amazing musicians for a three-month residency at Teach Furbo, a venue just a few miles from Galway. I was hopeful the band would stay together after the tour. It was also an opportunity for a reset after my relapse into depression.

Summer in Galway

By early April, the band began rehearsing in preparation for the trip. In addition, we did several gigs in New York which were a lot of fun. The music was of the highest standard, challenging me to rise to the level of musicianship of those around me. I decided to hold off any decision about school until the end of the Irish trip.

By June, it was time to head back to Ireland. The country, like the rest of the world, was in the midst of a recession and a gas (petrol) crisis. People queued up for hours just to get their ration of gas for the week. That made it difficult for many people to come see us but word quickly spread about this new band from America and people found ways to get to our shows.

The band was called Oceans Apart. Paddy Higgins, in addition to being a superb drummer, was a great storyteller and kept us entertained day and night. Our pedal steel guitar player Skip Krevens was over six feet tall and towered over the rest of us who struggled to reach five-foot six. In addition to being a prodigy musician, Skip was also as funny as hell and loved everything about Ireland. Chris Ebneth was a super-talented bass player and singer and was far and away the favorite with the young ladies in the audience.

With the exception of the drummer, everyone in the band was single, so there was a lot of romancing going on in the hotel attached to Teach Furbo where the band had their accommodations. The hotel was decrepit and on its last legs, but the cabaret room where we performed was perfect for our band. I stayed in the family home in Salthill, five miles from the venue.

There was a constant stream of visitors from the States to see the band thanks in large part to the big following Chris and Sean had in New York. Despite the gas crisis, by midsummer Oceans Apart developed a great reputation and it looked like another brush with fame was about to happen.

Dad and my sisters could see I had recovered well from my bout of depression earlier in the year, and it was great spending time with them. On several nights when I looked down at the audience, I saw Dad and a few of my sisters enjoying the music. Because I was there for several months, I was no longer the tourist or the visitor. It was like old times except I had a much better appreciation of how lucky I was to have such a loving family. I spent a lot of time sitting around our kitchen table with my sisters and some of the folks who had come from America to see the band just chatting and having a great laugh.

Word got around the country about this hot band from America making waves. We dressed different, we looked different and we were different. We took traditional Irish music places it had never been by adding all kinds of electronic synthesizers and rhythmic patterns. Once again, I had that rare indescribable feeling of knowing I was part of something incredibly special. It was that gestalt moment where the whole was bigger than the sum of the parts. We considered staying in Ireland to capitalize on the following and the momentum we had built up over the summer, but we decided against it given the commitments some members of the band had back in America.

I was convinced the band was going to be a great success, even more so than Rock & Roll Circus five years earlier. We all got along well and by the time the summer ended, the band was rock solid. I was devastated when I realized it was over.

Our final show was at the Castle Inn in the heart of Salthill. It was a great venue for live music and the place was jam packed. The energy in the room was electric from the moment we played that first note to the final chord of the last song. We got a standing ovation and two encores. The audience wouldn't let us off the stage.

I couldn't come to grips with the fact that the band had ended abruptly. After several months on this extraordinary journey, we were like family. Just like when my first band Spoonful broke up, it wasn't just the loss of the music, it was saying goodbye to my band family. I knew I could stay in touch with them, but it would never be the same as sharing a stage and experiencing the daily chemistry between us.

By mid-September, the rest of the band made their way back to the U.S. in the hope of reestablishing the careers and lives they left behind three months earlier. Musicians have their own language. Sometimes it's the silence between us that speaks volumes. As I bid farewell to each band member, we just nodded our heads. That simple gesture was an acknowledgment we shared something incredibly special. Despite the heartache, nothing can ever take those memories and shared experiences away.

Decision Time

In terms of my mental health, I was doing well most of the time. Every so often, the depression poked through, but I was better at recognizing the warning signs and taking action. I knew the breakup of the band and the uncertainty surrounding my future was going to be a challenge, but I was determined not to fall back into the darkness.

I needed time and space to think about all that had happened. I booked a holiday to Torremolinos in Spain's Costa Del Sol for a week, figuring it was away from both Ireland and America. It was somewhere neutral to get over my frustration and disappointment with the breakup of Oceans Apart. I also had a decision to make.

I took my guitar along on the trip. I was lonely for the first few days but quickly met some people from Ireland and the UK at a local bar. We had great music sessions in the afternoons on the beach and in the evenings at the bar. My emotions swung from each end of the pendulum as I did some serious soul searching. But overall, I had a great week, and by the time I landed at Dublin Airport a week later on a Saturday morning, I had a plan.

As luck would have it, Pope John Paul II was embarking on the first-ever papal visit to Ireland that same morning. My flight was the last to land before the Aer Lingus pontifical plane touched down on the tarmac. Ireland was abuzz in anticipation of the Pope's visit. As I left the airport on a crowded bus, we passed thousands of people making their way to an open-air mass at Phoenix Park in the center of Dublin. People were walking in all kinds of groups with signs and flags welcoming the Pope.

Some were praying and saying decades of the rosary in unison, others were singing hymns and the younger people were singing folk songs.

The bus dropped me off near the outskirts of Dublin on the main Galway Road. I began hitchhiking as there were no buses to Galway that early in the morning. It was still only 7 am and I was the lone person heading in the direction of Galway as the throngs of people made their way to the Pope's mass in Dublin.

I was tired and wondered if I'd ever get to Galway when a car pulled alongside and the driver offered me a ride. I got in only to recognize a friend I went to school with in St. Enda's. He was in the Irish Air Corps and part of the re-con group during the Pope's visit. Since there was nobody going in our direction and the cops weren't an issue given my friend's elevated status, we made great time and by 9 am he dropped me directly outside my home in Salthill.

I walked into the house expecting the family to be about their business, but they were all waiting for me with the welcome of the world. Within a few seconds, the kettle was on for the cuppa tea, which was a clear and direct signal they wanted to hear all the details of my Spanish adventure. There were hoots and hollers as I told them about seeing women on the beach topless and me getting burnt to a crisp that first day, most probably because I was enchanted to distraction by my topless neighbors. Nobody, including Dad, wanted to leave the kitchen table. He was literally heaving with laughter as I recounted my trip in detail.

I think it was then, with all of us sitting around the kitchen table, I realized I had re-established my relationship with Dad and my four sisters. I loved them for who they were then versus who they were five years ago when I left for America. Of course, they mourned the loss of Mam, but they adapted to a life without that wonderful lady guiding them through each day.

My sisters were in their early twenties when I left, a time of life when change happens rapidly. Now I was ready to embrace and celebrate those changes. The same was true of Dad. Of course, he missed Mam, but he was getting on with life.

During that summer, Dad and I had some great conversations. He enjoyed the music of Oceans Apart and kept telling my sisters, "Those lads are so feckin' professional." That was the utmost compliment from him. I think he was proud, but I don't think he was quite prepared for the news that would make him even prouder.

Pope John Paul II visited Galway on September 1, 1979, to celebrate an open-air youth mass at Ballybrit, the famed Galway horseracing track. Like Dublin, the town was buzzing. The gathering drew young people from all over Ireland and every corner of Europe.

The pubs stayed open late the night before the mass so people could have a wellness drink or two before embarking on the long walk to the racecourse. I went out with some friends to the local pub which had two sections, the Cottage Bar for the younger crowd and P.J. Flaherty's next to it for the older folks. Dad was having a few pints of Guinness in Flaherty's, so I left my friends for a few minutes to say hello. He was watching the TV and enjoying all the excitement. I asked him if he was going to see the Pope to which he quickly replied, "Why in the feckin' hell would I be going to see the Pope?" However, I learned the next day he stayed up most of the night and early morning shuttling senior citizens in his taxi for free to the raceway. It was his way of helping out.

"Dad, I've decided to start college in America in a few months," were the next words out of my mouth. He nearly fell off the bar stool. If I had handed him a million dollars, he wouldn't have been any happier. There was a broad smile on his face that seemed to last until I got back on the plane to America a few weeks later. I'm sure he was concerned how I was going to pay for college and adjust to it after seven years away from school. But I heard him say a million times, "An education is no burden to carry," and now his only son was about to gain that elusive education. I only wish Mam was sitting beside him in the pub to share in that beautiful moment.

After chatting with Dad, I headed home and met up with my sisters Carol and Toni and Pauline O'Carroll, a neighbor and dear friend of my sister Carol whom we often call our fifth sister. Our pilgrimage to Ballybrit, the site of the mass, started at three in the morning, so we had sandwiches packed and a flask of tea. My sisters and Pauline had an additional flask I didn't know about with something a bit stronger than the tea.

Getting half a million people to Ballybrit on Galway's small roads and the dirt paths in the vicinity of the racetrack was a logistical nightmare, but everyone was in good form and helping one another. The youth mass at the raceway was an extraordinary experience. It was one of those moments in life when you feel you're at the center of the universe. The racetrack was a sea of colors with school uniforms, community groups' banners, and thousands of flags representing organizations big and small.

It's hard to explain what it was like to see the sun break through the dark clouds over Galway with the Irish band the Chieftains playing their beautiful music to so many people. The crowd erupted in applause and screams of delight when John Paul II arrived next to the giant stage via the

Pope mobile—a big yellow contraption that allowed him to view the amazing vista from an elevated platform.

There was great hope that the Pope would have a significant impact on a world that seemed to be falling apart in the late '70s. The sectarian violence in Northern Ireland was at its worst, famine and starvation ravaged Africa, and the cold war was dangerously close to putting an end to our civilization.

The Catholic Church held the people of Ireland hostage since its independence in 1921 with its dogmatic teachings and antiquated practices that belonged to the dark ages. Just maybe, this man who possessed the charisma, optimism and hope that hadn't been seen since President John Fitzgerald Kennedy, might lift the permanent cloud that hung over our world. Most Irish households had a picture of Pope John XXIII and JFK hung side by side in their living rooms. Maybe this extraordinary man could provide some hope to the young people of Ireland, who were used to hearing absolute rubbish from the pulpit each Sunday when they attended mass with their families.

For that one Saturday in October, the Pope did shine a light but within a few years of his visit, the Catholic Church in Ireland was rocked by scandals involving child abuse and the horrors of the Magdalene Laundries, where unwed mothers were made to do slave labor and often forced to give up their children to adoption. The power of the Church in Ireland would never rise to the dizzying heights of that morning at the Galway racecourse in October 1979. It's hard to imagine that such a spectacular event marked the beginning of the end of the Catholic Church's domination in Ireland.

I returned to America shortly after the Pope's visit. Back in New York, I found plenty of work freelancing with different bands. I also performed solo shows for the first time in my career. I put an advertisement in the local Irish paper in New York and within weeks I was playing five nights a week. I experienced a great sense of independence performing on my own. During that period, I developed a banter with the audience. I've always enjoyed stand-up comedy—doing the solo shows gave me license to chat to the audience and develop a routine unique to me. I was still very shy but once I walked on stage, the other Seamus showed up.

Love and College Life

That October, I did a show on Long Island when I met Mary, a beautiful young lady from the Bronx. There have been more Marys in my life than you could shake a stick at. My mother was Mary, her mother was Mary. My dad's mother was Mary as was his grandmother. My first girlfriend in Ireland was Mary and there were more to come.

I stated dating this Mary and things got serious quickly. She was an only child. Her parents were from Ireland and she had spent many happy days there, so we had that love of my homeland in common. She enjoyed being around the Irish music scene. Her previous boyfriend was a musician, so we knew a lot of the same people. Like my mother, Mary was a nurse.

After several months dating, I proposed to Mary. It was altogether too short a courtship as I had little or no real dating experience. Also, I was about to start college. I didn't know it then, but the college experience would have a profound impact on all aspects of my life including my relationship with Mary. We planned on getting married in August of 1980.

I started college in January 16, 1980. It was cold, windy and dark when I got out of my car in the massive parking lot at Montclair State College in New Jersey. I asked myself what in the name of God was I doing? I was twenty-six and all the other students starting college were 18 or 19. I also had a major problem. I could barely read.

Reality hit home later that morning during my second class, "Intro to English Literature," when the professor handed out the syllabus with a reading list of seven books. That was six more than I had read in my life. I was distraught and started chatting to a guy sitting next to me. He could see I was in a bad way and said, "Don't worry, buddy, I've got you covered. There's a solution to your problem and it's called Cliff Notes. You'll find them for all the assigned books in the college bookstore. Don't worry too much about the book, just memorize the Cliff Notes."

Sure enough, I found the Cliff Notes along with the actual books. The Cliff Notes were basically a Reader's Digest version of each book. They summarized the plot, the main characters and the key points to remember for exam purposes. The notes were very much frowned upon by professors, but they became my best friend for my first few semesters at Montclair.

I found everything about college difficult. I was terrible at multiple choice tests as I had never taken one in Ireland. Also, I couldn't type, which was a major problem as all papers had to be typed. Thankfully, Mary was a great typist. She was incredibly supportive in every way during that first year. Thanks to Mary, my buddy who suggested the Cliff Notes and a professor who helped me develop a strategy for multiple choice exams, I managed to make it through that first semester with straight As. I had climbed my Mount Everest.

The day I got my results in the mail, I sent a letter to Dad telling him that in addition to passing all my exams, I made the Dean's List. I'm sure there were a few passengers in his taxi and some of his friends in his local pub Roddy Kelly's the day he received the letter from America, who were told the story of his son Seamus in America making the Dean's List with straight As. Mam and Dad dreamed that someday I would go back to college. That's why they insisted I pass the Leaving Certificate examination while fully supporting my dream of becoming a professional musician. By getting on the Dean's List, I felt I was standing up to my part of the bargain.

Even though Montclair was mainly a commuter college, I did enjoy the social aspect of meeting people from all over. But more importantly, I was like a sponge soaking up every opportunity I had to learn. My brain had awoken after it had been asleep for years. While music was still my passion, I had a new thirst for learning. I was mesmerized by the ideas of Socrates and Descartes and fascinated by the world of psychology which prompted me to examine some of the experiences that had shaped me, especially in my teen years. I read Hemingway and Dickens for the first time, finding much joy in the stories but also in the beauty of the words on the printed page.

I experienced a great sense of freedom and excitement at college but felt hemmed in by my relationship. Crossing over the George Washington Bridge on my way home to the Bronx was like crossing into a different world. The bridge was a metaphor for the divide between Mary and me. The bridge got longer with each passing day. Between college and my music schedule, Mary and I didn't have a lot of time to build our relationship. I knew we were rushing things.

The Jersey Shore

As the spring rolled around, my solo shows picked up momentum. I was asked to play a gig in Wildwood at the southernmost tip of the New Jersey Shore in a place called the Irishman's Café. It turned out to be a glorified audition. I walked into a cabaret-style room to find the average age of the audience somewhere between 65 and 85. I did a few Irish songs and two rock and roll tunes. Based on the muted reaction from the audience, I wasn't sure what they or the owner made of me. I was surprised to hear from him the following morning asking me to do a residency for the summer months, three nights a week, that would include accommodations and food. I jumped at the opportunity but told him I needed a few weeks off in August as I was getting married.

Wildwood was a large seaside resort consisting of a beautiful maze of inlets with a bay on one side and the Atlantic Ocean on the other. It was the summer get-away for people from all over Pennsylvania and New Jersey, but, in particular, the densely populated Philadelphia area, which was only two hours away. It had a boardwalk stretching over two miles punctuated by Morey's Pier amusement complex and various water parks. A tram car ran the length of the boardwalk, and fireworks lit up the sky each evening as the young and old enjoyed the beauty of the shore. Irish accents could be heard all over the boardwalk as young students came to live and work in Wildwood each summer on their J1 student visas.

Wildwood was broken into various sections: North Wildwood, a mix of ages and all kinds of entertainment venues; Wildwood, where the young folk gathered in the bars and clubs; and Wildwood Crest, which was more family-oriented and also home to many retirees.

The Irishman's Café was in North Wildwood and could accommodate 200 seated guests, with a big bar area off to the side. The stage was front and center. There was nowhere to hide if you were on the shy side.

My first show had about thirty people and I wondered if I made a mistake accepting the residency for the entire summer. But each week, the crowd doubled in size. By mid-July, I walked on stage every night to over two hundred people. I got to know the audience members since most of them were regulars.

Johnny Carson was the king of late-night TV with The Tonight Show in the 1980s. He had a remarkable way of engaging his guests without ever telling a joke. I rarely missed his nightly show. He had a profound influence on me as I developed my stage persona.

Each morning, I read the papers to catch the local news. I learned about the schools the audience members attended, their sports teams and any social or political drama going on in the Philadelphia or Wildwood area. I learned that folks from Philadelphia loved to make fun of the French Canadians who came to Wildwood in droves early August. They were known for their lack of swim attire on the beach, which made them an easy target. I familiarized myself with the sports teams such as the Eagles, the 76ers, the Flyers and the key college rivalries.

Each night, before playing my first song, I sat on a bar stool and talked to the audience telling stories, making fun of the different Catholic schools and the Philly sport teams. I also talked about what was in the papers that day, much like Carson did during his monologue at the beginning of The Tonight Show. I think the older folks wondered how a young fella from Ireland could know so much about their world. I was honing my craft.

I enjoyed every minute on stage at the Irishman's Café and made some wonderful friends along the way. In particular, I became great friends with Tom and Gerry Caufield—two of the kindest and funniest people I've ever known. They provided me with a great education on the Philadelphia scene musically and socially. They took me around Wildwood to the various venues and introduced me as a mini celebrity to many lovely people. We became lifelong friends.

The owner of the Irishman's Café was Michael Garvin, a lovely man in his early forties, who left the priesthood after 20 years to marry his wife Mary—I'm not making this up. Mary left the convent where she was a nun around the same time, also after a twenty-year stint. Mary and Michael were from well-known conservative Catholic families. It was a love story in the eyes of many and a scandal in the eyes of a few.

I had my own room in their apartment above the bar. I became part of their family over that summer. We had great times talking about the characters we dealt with each night during my performances. The bar was getting busier with each passing day. They knew I was responsible for bringing in the crowds, especially earlier in the week, on what should have been quiet nights and they appreciated it.

Parallel Lives

Mary and I were married in August. Because of the all-too-short courtship, my family in Ireland had not met her. In the run-up to the wedding, I felt very alone and unsure of what I was doing because I knew we were rushing things. I considered calling the wedding off but worried about how that would impact Mary.

My sister Carol came out from Ireland for the wedding and that helped lift my spirits. She was a great support during that time, but I didn't share my concerns with her.

The actual wedding went off without a hitch. Everyone had a great time. Afterwards we went straight to Wildwood at the Jersey Shore, as I promised Mike Garvin I would do two shows at the Irishman's Café before heading to Ireland on our official honeymoon. Mary and I had a great time at the shore, and the doubts I had before the wedding began to fade, at least temporarily.

The trip to Ireland also went well. We were there for my sister Toni's wedding. My family all loved Mary and got along with her from the moment they set eyes on her. We had some lovely times exploring Ireland together. I met Mary's extended family in County Cork and enjoyed their company. They welcomed me with open arms.

Upon our return to New York, I went back to college. Things were good and I threw myself back into my studies. I was very fortunate to come across a great teacher at Montclair, Francine Shaw. She could have walked straight out of a day-time soap opera set. She was glamorous and always dressed up for class complete with full makeup and an elaborate hairstyle. She had a wonderful aura about her.

There was a lot of reading involved in her class, so I thought it wise to let her know about my reading difficulties. While my reading had improved, it was still my biggest weakness. Ironically, her class was focused on teaching English to young children. The books she assigned were academic in nature and didn't have Cliff Notes so I couldn't fake it. She asked me to come to her office the next afternoon.

She spent an hour a day with me over a period of weeks showing me how to read and how to focus on what was important in the text. Within a month, I was reading a book a week and I was able to remember the content, something I could never do before. Not only did Francine Shaw make my years at Montclair State College easier, but she also unlocked the door for me to read newspapers so I was more informed on the events of the day. I was also able to manage my way through books that previously eluded me. To this day, I'm an avid reader and that skill has provided me many great opportunities over the years. Learning to read properly also spurred a desire to write, something that had never entered my mind prior to meeting the beautiful Francine Shaw.

Mary could not have been more supportive during those college years, but part of me felt I just wasn't present. It's hard to explain looking back on it, but it was as if my life was on hold. Much of this had to do with my mental state. It wasn't quite depression, but something wasn't right. I was turning inward again, and Mary and I were growing further apart. I was existing rather than living. We were living parallel lives.

During my third year of college, I damaged my voice. During my shows, I was fine for the first few songs but then I had a sensation of choking and not being able to get enough air. Bar owners, staff and audience members noticed something was drastically wrong. One owner, Terry Connaughton, from the Riverdale Steak House in the Bronx, took me aside during a break and said, "You know how much we all love you here at the Riverdale Steak House, Seamus, but we are worried about you. Your voice is not the same and it's impacting your show. Maybe you need a break for a while." I didn't know how to react. My body stiffened hearing those words from Terry. If my biggest supporter was telling me I was in trouble, what were the other owners thinking? I knew Terry was looking out for me. I had worked so hard to build my reputation, but each time I walked on stage with my voice the way it was, that reputation suffered.

A top specialist in New York examined my vocal cords and the only thing he could put my condition down to was utter exhaustion and stress. Doing at least five shows a week while attending college fulltime was taking a toll. He suggested I stop singing for at least six months and whisper rather than talk. I left the doctor's Park Avenue office feeling completely numb. Part of me wished there was a concrete diagnosis so I could know what was wrong. I wondered if I'd ever sing again, or if I'd be able to talk to an audience from the stage. I finally found a way to break with my shyness and communicate with people but felt it was being taken away from me—possibly forever. I feared I'd fall back into full-blown depression as my mood got darker with each day.

Not being able to perform meant my income vanished overnight. I took out my calendar and cancelled every show for the next six months. Financially, Mary and I were okay as she had a steady paycheck from nursing, and we lived modestly in an apartment in the Bronx. As always, she was supportive and never made me feel like I was letting her or myself down. But at a time when we should have been putting money away for a house, I felt I put us both in a difficult situation.

Flanagan's on First

Prior to losing my voice, I had a bass player/singer, Barry Lynch, with me for some shows. He was super talented and a pleasure to work with. We became dear friends. I played golf with Sean Fleming one afternoon and said in my new whisper voice, "Sean, why don't I play guitar with you but you also need to take my bass player Barry Lynch and, I can't sing or talk for at least six months." He laughed at my crazy idea but said he would think about it. Sean called me a few days later and agreed to my nutty proposal, thus beginning another chapter on my musical journey. Joining up with Sean took the financial pressure away and most importantly, it got me back on stage.

Barry, Sean and I sounded good as a three-piece band. Since I couldn't sing, I focused exclusively on my lead guitar playing, something I had neglected as a solo artist. Barry's incredible voice was a perfect match for Sean in terms of harmonies and he also took the pressure off him by singing several songs throughout the show. We played four nights a week in Flanagan's on First Avenue in Manhattan. Sean had been there for years and had a huge following. Every night was a packed house.

Flanagan's was an extraordinary venue. Walking in from the street, there was a long bar on the right-hand side and to the left a cabaret room with red leather booths and Tiffany-style lighting. It's hard to know what makes a venue special, but whatever it is, Flanagan's had it. A large part of the magic was the staff. Each bartender had their own following. The waitresses knew every customer by name and the maître d', Sammy O' Connor from Belfast, never forgot a name or a face and made whoever walked through the doors feel special.

Two bands performed at Flanagan's each night, alternating shows from 9 pm 'til 3 am. We gave it our all each night on stage and the breaks between shows allowed us to interact with the audience on a personal level. Sean is a master entertainer and I learned so much by just watching how he grabbed the audience and took them on a different journey each evening. Now that I was on lead guitar duty four nights a week, my playing improved dramatically.

After a year playing in Flanagan's, Sean partnered with some friends and bought a bar on 86th Street between First and Second Avenues and named it Fleming's. The place had a wonderful cabaret room that could seat about eighty people. There was a downstairs bar area that could accommodate 150 or so and most of them could still see the music in the cabaret room. It was an exciting time for Sean, finally having his own place. We moved shop to Fleming's playing four nights a week and much of the Flanagan's crowd followed.

The Graduate

It was a busy time for me playing four nights a week at Fleming's and attending college five days a week. I got by on very little sleep. Sean also travelled to Washington and Philadelphia for shows so sometimes I had to commute back hundreds of miles for an 8 am class in New Jersey. I didn't care as I loved playing with Sean and I knew I had less than a year left of college.

When I started at Montclair, I was a music therapy major but I switched to music education as I felt it was a better match for me. As part of the degree, I had to student teach. I was placed at a school in New Jersey and loved the teaching experience. It was tough work since I was still taking classes in the evening at Montclair, playing music with Sean Fleming in New York and student teaching five day a week.

I was also preparing for a classical guitar recital, a requirement for graduation. I practiced at least three hours every day and during my breaks at Fleming's, I went downstairs to the liquor room and played guitar. At college, I grabbed the guitar any free minute I had.

The classical guitar is completely different from playing electric guitar and it allowed me to hear music in another way. It was like having an orchestra in my hands. By my final year at Montclair, I developed my own style of playing. I enjoyed learning the classical repertoire that included the works of Francisco Tárrega, Heitor Villa-Lobos and Mauro Giuliani. Much like how learning to read opened my mind to words on a printed page, the classical guitar opened my ears to a whole new world of music.

I was surprised and delighted when my sister Maura came out from Ireland to attend my graduation recital. She was always an ardent

152

supporter of my crazy career and never doubted I'd succeed in music. On the night of the recital, she brought my Aunt Nora along making the evening even more special. Mary, as always, was there to support me.

When the day of the recital finally came, I was terrified before going on stage. To this day, I get nervous in front of an audience despite having done close to 8,000 shows during my career. But getting up in front of the faculty, students, my friends and family at Montclair was different. For the recital, I sat on a stool resting the guitar on my knee, but my entire body was shaking so much that the guitar felt like it was jumping up and down. After a few pieces, the nerves settled, and the recital went much better than I could have hoped for.

I got a standing ovation after the final piece. I was thrilled and felt an enormous sense of relief. I couldn't believe I made it through the hour-long performance—I was walking on air—I did it. Four years of blood, sweat and tears paid off. I already knew I was graduating with high honors on the academic side but getting a giant hug and a thumbs-up from my guitar teacher was the final seal of approval.

Immediately following the recital, I had a small reception for friends and family in a room behind the auditorium. My Aunt Nora was beaming, Maura couldn't control the tears and Mary was delighted to see the long hours of practice pay off.

My teacher Howard Greenblatt—a lovely man and great guitar player—was very complimentary after my performance saying I had the potential to make a career playing the classical guitar if I chose to do so. He particularly enjoyed my banter with the audience and some of the liberties I took with the classical repertoire, something frowned upon in the world of classical music. A career as a classical guitarist was not my goal, and despite the encouragement from Greenblatt, I was well aware I fell fairly low on the totem pole of classical guitar players. But stretching myself and getting to the level I did helped shape my music career ever since. I had come a long way from that first classical guitar lesson at the American Institute of Guitar after arriving in America in 1975.

A month later, Dad, along with my sister Geraldine, came out from Ireland for my actual graduation. We weren't sure until the very last moment if he was actually going to come. Dad was terrified about getting on the plane for the six-and-a-half-hour journey to America. But my sisters told him how much it would mean to have him there. He relented at the last minute and stepped on the plane at Shannon after a few glasses of whisky.

Dad loved watching American detective shows on TV where New York City was often portrayed as a gray concrete jungle. He was shocked to see the lovely tree-lined streets of Woodlawn in the Bronx where Mary and I lived. I found him a local pub within walking distance of our apartment, a place he could relax during his visit. A friend of Dad's, Tadhg Murphy, who years earlier worked with him in the post office in Galway, now lived in New York. Tadhg had great time for Dad and met up with him a few times at the pub, making sure he felt welcome.

After I walked into the football stadium at Montclair State in my cap and gown for my graduation ceremony, I made eye contact with Dad and Ger. It was a moment in time to be cherished—an image etched in my mind forever. Dad waved his hand in recognition. Dad's job was done, his son finally had that prized college degree, and not only that, but he also graduated magna cum laude.

It was lovely having Dad in New York. He got to experience the world that I lived in since leaving Ireland nine years earlier. We took the Circle Line boat tour around Manhattan. It was a spectacular day and Dad was in his element as we sailed up the East River passing the UN's iconic towering white building. He was emotional as we passed the Statue of Liberty and Ellis Island. What was it was like for his sisters, Rita and Nora, who arrived by boat to the port of New York shortly after Ellis Island closed? Dad was just a boy when they left their home in Kerry.

We also brought Dad to Fleming's where he saw me perform with Sean and Barry. The staff fussed over him all night long making him feel special and he got to know my other family. Another high point of that week was seeing him enjoy time with his sister Nora. They talked for hours as if they had been living down the road from each other all their lives, often breaking into fluent Gaelic, the language they grew up with and one they both cherished. It was wonderful to hear the beautiful inflections and the lilt in their voices as they went from a quiet voice to belly-aching laughter. Dad had that same priceless bond with his sisters I have with mine.

Dad was glad to get back on that Aer Lingus plane after his week in New York. Other than a weekend in London, the trip to New York was the only time he had been away from Ireland. He was a homebody, but according to my sisters, when they gathered in the pub upon his return for the traditional meeting and information sharing, it was the most animated they had seen him in years. He recounted everything he had experienced in America in vivid detail, but what stood out in his mind was the tree-lined streets of the Bronx. He couldn't get over it.

Saddest of Times

While I was delighted to be done with college, I felt a void in my life. Things were not great with my marriage and I wasn't ready to have children. Already feeling confused about where I was in life, I got a call from my sister Geraldine telling me Dad had a terrible accident at home and suffered deep burns on his lower back. Initially it looked like he would make a recovery but then the girls said that I might want to come home to see him. A chill went through me. Dad was indestructible; he had been through a lot in life, but always came out on the other side. I couldn't comprehend a life without him.

As it turned out, I was playing a show in Italy with Sean Fleming a week after Ger called. Immediately after the show at the Excelsior Hotel in Rome, I flew to Ireland. I went straight from Dublin Airport to St. Stephan's Hospital, arriving late in the evening. My sisters Carol and Toni met me at the burn unit and warned me that it might be hard to see Dad the way he was.

But nothing prepared me for what I saw. Dad was in a bad way. He was surprised to see me and a broad smile came across his face, but it was clear he was in terrible pain. I made believe that I just popped in because I was on my way back to America from Rome. I asked how he was doing, and he said, "Jim, this is my crucifixion." This coming from a man I never heard complain about a pain in his life. Those words felt like a knife twisting around in my heart.

I walked out of the hospital ward into the chilly October night air. Without saying anything to my sisters, I circled around the hospital courtyard several times and burst into tears. I sobbed uncontrollably for ten minutes, my entire body heaving. It pained me to see a man who had helped so many people during his lifetime suffer. He didn't deserve this. I knew deep inside he wouldn't recover. Carol and Toni let me come to grips with my grief. When the time was right, they walked over and hugged me tight.

Three of my sisters had young children back in Galway. Between them, they did shifts making sure Dad had someone by his bedside every day. All four sisters stepped up to the plate but it was incredibly hard for them as Galway was over 120 miles away and the roads in the middle of winter were not great. There were moments when it looked like Dad might pull through, but as I left to go back to America, I began to face the reality of a life without my hero.

I came back to Ireland a few weeks later to help my sisters out and provide some emotional support. Dad was slowly slipping away and didn't recognize me. That was hard, but I was glad to be there for him and especially for my siblings, who were exhausted mentally and physically. I said my goodbye to Dad before heading back to America. It was difficult getting on the plane at Dublin Airport.

New Year's Eve was always a big night in New York. The Sean Fleming Band was making some serious waves. In addition to the New Year's Eve show at Fleming's, immediately afterwards, we were to perform at a high-profile gig for the staff of MTV. It was a big deal.

On December 29, 1985, I got the dreaded call from my sister Geraldine saying Dad had passed. I knew the call was coming, but it still hurt. I loved my Dad more than words can ever express. He never fully recovered from the passing of Mam ten years earlier. I believe, once I graduated in 1984, he felt his job was done. All five of his children were on their way.

Since I had been home to Ireland twice to see Dad in the two months since the accident, my sisters and I agreed in advance of Dad's passing I wouldn't go home for the funeral. But after getting off the phone with Geraldine, I felt uncomfortable with that decision. For some reason, the image of Dad's casket being carried into the church in Galway without his only son present didn't feel right. I needed closure; I wanted to say a final goodbye to Dad.

Thanks to a dear friend, Ella O'Sullivan, who worked with Aer Lingus, I was booked at the very last minute on a flight to Dublin and a return flight to get me back in time for the shows with Sean Fleming on New Year's Eve. I arrived unannounced to the hotel in Dublin where my sisters were staying. The four of them were sitting around a table having breakfast. I knew immediately from the look on their shocked faces I made the right decision by coming home. There was no hiding our emotions. The tears were flowing and there were long hugs and smiles of relief. We were all together now and that's what our lovely Dad would have wanted. The girls were under enormous pressure for two solid months seeing Dad slip away under such difficult and sad circumstances. They had to keep a brave face for their young children who kept asking about their YaYa (the name they had given to their grandfather). Now we could grieve together.

The five of us went to the morgue to see our father one last time. It was hard but it gave us closure. Shortly afterwards, we headed back to Galway in a procession of seven cars following the hearse with Dad's casket. The hearse driver let me sit in the passenger seat. It was only when we reached the outskirts of Galway, the city Dad loved so much, when it fully hit me this was his final journey.

The church in Salthill was packed when we arrived at dusk. I was surprised by the number of young people who showed up. A lot of them were friends of mine and my sisters, but others were people whose lives Dad had touched over the years with his kindness and generosity. There was a line of taxis parked outside the church. Dad was a big part of the growth of the business in Galway, so all the taxi drivers showed up to pay their respect, as did people who worked with him in the post office and folks he served with in the army.

My sisters and I were at the front of the church next to the casket as people came up and introduced themselves and explained how they knew Dad. I often wonder about the wisdom of that tradition, especially when one is experiencing such grief at the loss of a loved one, but I found it comforting to have the support of so many. It allowed us to get a glimpse at the lives Dad had touched in some way during his 69 years.

That night, we gathered in our home in Salthill with friends and family in celebration of Dad's life. He once remarked after a few whiskies that he wished he was a better Catholic. I remember thinking he was more of a Christian than most people I knew. When others were going to mass every day, often putting on show so that everybody knew they were a "good" church-going Catholic, Dad, like our Mam, spent his life helping others. In Dad's case, sometimes it was not taking a cab fare from an old lady, giving money to those in need or just listening to the struggles of one of his passengers and sharing some of his wisdom. He never expected thanks for his kind acts. To me, that's what we should all strive for in life.

The funeral took place the following morning. It was incredibly sad. I played a classical guitar piece, "Romanza," after the homily. Then, I placed my hand on the coffin and said goodbye to Dad. My heart was broken as I looked back at my sisters as they did their best to control their tears.

I walked out of the church halfway through the service into a waiting car driven by Andy McEntee, the drummer from Rock & Roll Circus. Andy drove like a Formula One driver so I could make a flight from Shannon Airport that would get me back to New York in time for my shows in Fleming's and MTV. As we drove to the airport, I was thinking of my sisters who were by then at the graveyard as Dad's remains were placed next to Mam's.

Like Mam, Dad gave my sisters and I the gift of unconditional love. It's the greatest gift a parent can give a child. That love is like a bottomless well you can draw on throughout your life. I've been to the well many times.

Ten hours later, I walked on stage at Fleming's. I knew Dad would want me to get back to work. But my world had changed. Something happens when you lose both your parents. You look at your life through a different lens and become acutely aware of your own mortality. I began to question everything: who I was as a person, my music and especially my marriage.

Beginning and an End

When Dad passed, I was teaching music a few days a week at Saint Jerome's, a Catholic school in the South Bronx that served the predominantly Black and Hispanic community. The children, ranging in age from 10 to 14, were fun and full of energy and mischief. The school principal was an exceptional human being. All she cared about was providing those kids a great education in a safe and welcoming environment. Some of the students came from broken homes and their lives were not always easy. The principal treated me so well, as did all the staff, and the children loved the music. I brought the guitar into class each day and often let the children play. For many, it was the first time in their lives holding a musical instrument. I loved watching their eyes light up as they touched the strings and heard the sound reverberate through the classroom. It reminded me of the rare moments of joy at St. Edna's when I had that similar experience many years earlier.

I also taught one day a week at another Catholic school, St. Alexander's in Mamaroneck, one of the wealthiest suburbs north of New York City. In many ways, it was the polar opposite to the South Bronx. The kids were mainly White and came from predominantly wealthy families. But, as with the children at St. Jerome's, they were also beautiful.

The teaching was exhausting as I had two days a week in the South Bronx and one day at Mamaroneck. In St. Alexander's, I had a big auditorium/gymnasium as my classroom. I used the gym equipment and theatre props to set up elaborate musical games for the students. Each day we created a new adventure. I did a Christmas concert at the school, the first in many years. For most of the students, it was their first time on stage, and it was like they were performing at Carnegie Hall. It wasn't exactly Mr. Holland's Opus, but they were special times for me and, I hope, for the students.

By late spring, I knew my marriage was coming to an end. Mary and I had been together for over five years. We shared many happy times, but had grown apart. I moved out in June of 1986. It was a sad time. The end of our marriage was difficult for both of us, but it was also hard for our families and mutual friends.

My sisters were shocked and disappointed and feared I was making a terrible mistake. Part of the problem was I kept things to myself. Everything was bottled up inside ready to explode. College had changed me and I had all kinds of ideas going around in my head and felt I couldn't share them with Mary. She was a super smart lady but we had different interests. I suppressed my uncertainly about my marriage for years and it took a toll. I was trying to be what people wanted me to be rather than who I was.

The breakup was further complicated as I was becoming increasingly well-known because of the music. Rumors began to fly and people took sides. I worried about Mary, as I still cared deeply for her. There were days when I felt I should try harder to make it work but, deep down, I believed it was the right time for both of us to move on.

At the time of the breakup, MTV was showing continued interest in the band and Sean found investors to fund an all-original album. We recorded in some of New York's best studios with the famed Elliott Randall as producer. He had done the iconic guitar work for Steely Dan's "Reelin' in the Years." It was an incredible opportunity for us. What should have been the most exciting and exhilarating time in my life,

162

recording with some world class musicians in New York's famous Clinton Studios, was clouded by the heartache I experienced with the breakup of my marriage. The entire recording process is just a haze in my memory bank.

I stayed with some dear friends who lived in Queens following the separation with Mary. They were kind and gave me space to deal with what had happened and to contemplate what lay ahead. Each day, I experienced a range of emotions. One minute, I felt a weight off my chest knowing that I had made the hardest decision of my life. I was excited to face each day not waiting for my life to begin. The next, I wondered if I had made an awful mistake.

Several very close friends cut off all communications with me. They felt I was the bad guy. It's hard to blame them as I hadn't shared my struggles with anyone prior to the break-up. Losing some dear friends during that time was hard and added to the pain I felt.

After three weeks with my friends in Queens, I moved into a boarding house in Manhattan, not far from Fleming's. I had a tiny room with one small window with two metal bars on it. The house was a sad and lonely place. Like me, most of the residents were dealing with some kind of trauma. Each face I passed in the bleak hallway had a story to tell but few words were spoken. It was all in our eyes and body movement.

A Friend in Need

After a month in the rooming house, I went for a walk one gorgeous evening on the upper East Side of Manhattan to get away from the dreariness of my dark room. I passed opulent apartment buildings with doormen dressed in perfectly tailored outfits. I saw people of all ages on the streets and hearing their talking and laughter made me wonder if I would ever be like them. I envied the joy they were experiencing, even with the simple things in life, like walking down the street on a summer's evening.

During my walk, I came across a garbage truck with the driver trying to change a huge tire. I was watching him maneuver the tire into position when I ran into someone I knew from Fleming's. His name was Robert Hockberg. Rob was a big fan of the band and we got talking. I told him about the breakup of my marriage and in passing I mentioned my living situation. Without a moment's hesitation he said, "Yo, buddy, that sucks. I have an extra room in my apartment a few blocks from here. Let me talk to my roommate and see if we can help you out." It seemed too good to be true. I knew Rob was well intentioned, but I didn't get my hopes up.

Rob was on his way to play guitar with some friends and invited me along. We played for a few hours and then to my surprise he said, "Yo buddy, let's go back to my apartment and talk to my roommate Dave about that room. It's hard seeing you like this." It was 1 am and I wasn't sure if this was the right time to wake his roommate but that's what Rob did. Having been abruptly awoken from a deep sleep, Dave, listened to my story and said, "I'm good, let's do it." My jaw dropped. Could this be real?

It was a beautiful second-floor apartment on 82nd Street between Lexington and Park Avenue. The building had a spacious lobby and one of those old ornate, dark wooden elevators you see in the movies. The apartment was incredibly spacious by New York standards. The old Park Avenue apartments often had a maid's room complete with a tiny bathroom. Rob and Dave used that room for storage. They pulled out some of the furniture so I could take a proper look at it. At 2 am, Rob said, "It's yours buddy if you want it." I was in shock. He knew I was struggling financially and said, "Just pay $200 a month until you get back on your feet—we can increase the rent a bit then."

I don't think my feet hit the ground on my way back to the rooming house. When I woke the next morning after a fitful sleep, I wondered if I dreamt what happened the night before. I was expecting a call from Rob saying maybe it wasn't a good idea after all. Two days later, I moved my few personal belongings into my new apartment. Rob and Dave cleaned out my room and spruced it up for me. It was an extraordinary act of kindness for someone they didn't know, other than seeing me perform on stage at Fleming's.

Fleming's and the Drink

Fleming's was in its third year of operations at the time of my separation. It was the place to be seen on the Upper East Side of New York. There were lines outside every Friday and Saturday night. I'm not sure what it was, but once you walked into the bar, you entered another world. The bartenders were all from Ireland and at the top of their game. They made eye contact with each customer when they entered Fleming's and by the time they made it to the bar, a drink was waiting along with a warm welcome. The waitresses were equally hospitable, making sure every customer had everything they needed to make their evening something to remember.

The staff at Fleming's were one big family. Most of them were ten years younger than me. We hung out together and watched out for one another. We all knew something special was happening, with the crowds getting bigger with each passing week. As I went through the divorce proceedings, the staff knew I was hurting and were incredibly supportive and protective of me.

I was thirty-two years old and I had never taken a drink in my life. There was a lot of drinking in my family growing up and it had a devastating impact on me. I was well aware of the damage that excessive drinking could do and was always scared to start for fear it would impact my fragile mental state.

One wet and dreary afternoon, I went to the dentist in midtown Manhattan for a bridge impression. The dentist had a hard time making things work and I was in the chair for well over two hours. I left there feeling like a pin cushion after multiple doses of Novocain. I needed to sit down and have a cup of coffee to settle my nerves. I couldn't find a coffee shop so I ducked into Barrington's bar and restaurant thinking the bartender would surely give me a cup of coffee. I was out of luck. "Sorry bud, no coffee," said the bartender. I could see the coffee pot behind him, which pissed me off. I said, "Give me an Irish coffee then." I had two of them in quick succession and got back on the New York subway feeling happy. I felt like singing. I forgot about the dentist, the separation and impending divorce, and felt an inner glow and a tingling sensation that reached every cell of my body. It was a feeling I never experienced before—I was intoxicated for the first time in my life.

Every Thursday evening, a wealthy businessman named Gerry came into Fleming's. Before the band even got on stage, he insisted on buying us a bottle of Dom Pérignon. The waitresses loved this, as Sean Fleming didn't drink much champagne, our bass player was a beer drinker and, of course, I didn't drink. The waitresses got to drink most of the $100-a-bottle of bubbly. That changed after my experience with the Irish coffees. It didn't take long for me to start chugging the champagne. It made me feel a bit different. I was getting buzzed. After my initial drink, it was time to broaden my horizons and thus began a love affair with brandy.

Joining the Party

I was known as the quiet man in Fleming's. I was always reading a book or playing a guitar. I loved hanging out with everyone but I was never part of the conversation. I had plenty to say but felt nobody would find my input interesting. That changed as the champagne and my new best friend, brandy (or, to be specific, Rémy Martin VSOP) took effect. The quiet man went through a dramatic change over a period of a few months. I began to express my opinions on everything from sports to politics and, to my surprise, people listened. I often held court in Fleming's at the end of the evening, telling stories about growing up in Galway and opening up for bands like Thin Lizzy.

As the months progressed, I enjoyed the single life once again. On the nights I wasn't working, I was out on the town with the staff at Fleming's or hanging with my roommates Rob and Dave.

I was also spending a lot of time with Ginny, a beautiful girl from New Jersey who was a regular at Fleming's. We talked for hours on every subject under the sun. She was incredibly smart and challenged me to engage in well-informed conversation on everything from history and politics to books and family. We both loved New York and spent many days walking its avenues and streets talking and laughing and inhaling the sights and sounds of the city. We became very close and, over time, fell deeply in love.

With the passing of Dad and the trauma of the separation, I had no interest in food and lost close to forty pounds. While it wasn't the ideal way to lose weight, I did need to trim down. Chris Bishop, who recently joined the band as our new bass player, was an extraordinary musician, a super nice guy and a dapper dresser. He had worked with Robert Palmer for years. We hit it off immediately. For the first time in years, I paid attention to what I was wearing and consulted with Chris about my clothing choices. Being that I now weighed 155 pounds instead of 195, I had options other than baggy shirts and pants to conceal my bulging belly.

Several months after meeting Ginny, I passed a hair salon on Lexington Ave and through the large plate-glass window recognized one of the hairdressers who was a regular at Fleming's. I waved to her and she signaled me to come inside. I should have known from her name, Ice, and from her spiked blond hair, she was not your normal hairdresser. I walked out of the salon two hours later with spiked blonde highlights similar to Ice's, pointing straight into the air thanks to copious amount of that Aqua Net Extra Super Hold hair spray. Ginny was not amused when she saw me later that evening. In fact, she was horrified.

Not long after moving into Manhattan, I felt I needed to give something back to the community. I was lucky to have a good paying job doing what I loved and my roommates, through their kindness, helped me get back on my feet.

I had a bar-owner friend, Ronan Downs, who ran boat rides and had special dinners during the holidays collecting money for those less fortunate. After way too many drinks at his bar one night, I suggested we form an organization to get the young Irish immigrants more involved in the broader New York community. We wrote the mission statement on a napkin in his bar that simply said, "Helping those in need." We called our organization Celtic Care and over the course of several years raised over $250,000 for the New York homeless.

I always felt like I was on the outside looking in at social gatherings, be it at family or public gatherings. That began to change. All of a sudden, I was one of the cool people. I was playing with an amazing band, the pot belly was gone, and my pageboy haircut was replaced by a blonde highlighted mullet. I was invited to parties, or out to watch football games with friends, and for the first time in my life, girls were taking a second look at me. I even had a little groupie following at Fleming's.

Ginny was doing a master's degree at Johns Hopkins in Baltimore, so we saw less of each other. As I emerged from the fog of the lengthy divorce, I made up for my quiet years in droves. I went out most of my nights off from the band. Because of the popularity of Fleming's, there was no problem getting into any club. I just had the bartender call in advance and my name was at the door of the China Club, the Cat Club, Tramps or anywhere I wanted to go.

I went out to dinner on a regular basis with friends as very little cooking was done in the apartment. It was a new experience for me. Prior to that, eating was more of a chore, but now I looked forward to trying new foods and the experience of talking to people over dinner, something that had never appealed to me before.

Months after I started drinking, there was a birthday party for one of the Fleming's staff at a bar a few blocks from where I lived. Every time I looked around, my brandy snifter was full to the brim with Rémy Martin. The energy in the room was pure electric with everyone in great spirits. At one point in the evening as we listened to Frank Sinatra's "I Get a Kick out of You," we all piled into the tiny men's bathroom just to see how many of us would fit. It was pure honest-to-goodness innocent fun and silliness. At 3 am, I began the five-block walk home to my apartment. I was unsteady on my feet and kept banging into the walls of apartment buildings on my way. I made it to my building and spent at least twenty minutes trying to figure out why the key wouldn't turn. I finally realized I was on the wrong floor of the building. I no sooner made it to the bedroom of my apartment when the room started spinning uncontrollably and I threw up all over my bed. It was the first clear indication that the drink and I were not a great combination.

It was around this time that I discovered Eamonn Doran's, a New York institution within the drinking community. It was an extraordinary place and it wasn't uncommon to go there on a Monday at midnight and emerge with a hundred fellow revelers at 5 am the next morning. Sean Smyth, the bartender, was a gentle soul but didn't take crap from anybody. We quickly became great buddies. Most weekends, I left Fleming's at 3 am after getting off stage and hopped in a taxi for the ten-minute ride to Eamonn's. If I made it there by 3:30 am, I was allowed to stay until closing which was never earlier than 5 am. Next door was the Green Derby, owned by Terry O'Neill, the same owner as Fleming's. Of course, I got the royal treatment there and developed a great friendship with the bartender Danny McDonald.

Most Fridays and Saturdays after the Fleming's gig were spent shuffling between Eamonn's and the Derby. It was not unusual to be sitting next to a celebrity in Eamonn's. One night, Sean, the bartender, moved my drink and me away from Richard Harris saying afterwards, "You don't need to be listening to his crap tonight, Seamus, he's talking shite." On another evening, I was across from Sinéad O'Connor. She had performed a big concert in Manhattan, but she was just one of the crowd, no different from me or the cast of characters who frequented Doran's and the Derby.

Eamonn Doran, the owner, was a big round Santa Claus of a man and kind to everyone he set eyes on. He gave a start to many who emigrated from Ireland in the '70s and '80s. He reminded me of Dad in that he was always helping those less fortunate, often at his own expense. Eamonn had that wonderful gift that when he walked into the room, he became the center of attention, even though it was the last thing in the world he wanted. The rich, the not-so-rich and the famous loved him. His wife, Claire, was equally kind and played a major role in keeping the business afloat. The Dorans had two sons, Eddie and Dermott. Eddie was the more gregarious of the two, often getting into all kinds of tight spots. Dermott was the more artistic, but both loved the music and were always very supportive of me and my music. I believe I slept in Eamonn's one night after being over-served by Sean. Eddie told me to make sure to slam the door after me when I was ready to go home.

Another Fifteen Minutes

Fleming's was so busy on weekends I had to have the bouncer lift my guitar over the crowds crushing up against the bar just to get to the stage. MTV was just coming into its own in the mid-eighties, and one of the top executives, Rick Krim, lived around the corner. He was a regular and brought in some of the MTV staff, in particular, the vice president, Les Garland. Les was an energetic character and loved our band. I got a call from Rick saying that Les was very interested in doing something with us. Les asked Rick to set up a meeting at MTV's headquarters in Times Square. Sean Fleming, Chris Bishop and myself arrived down all decked out in our stage clothes with our hair held together by the Aqua Net hair spray we all used but wouldn't admit it. We were ushered into Garland's plush office. He basically said he would like to set us up with a record company. At this point in time, MTV was the only game in town and, for a record company, a phone call from Les Garland was like God calling. Any label would have taken us on, like us our not, just to get their other artists on MTV's video rotation.

Sadly, the meeting with MTV didn't go well. After much back and forth, there were concerns about Garland's direction for the band and we couldn't come to an understanding. The meeting ended abruptly, as did our opportunity to partner with MTV.

The Postman

It might have been the train wreck with MTV or the fact that my girlfriend Ginny had completed her master's degree in Baltimore, but all of a sudden, I had the urge to go back to college. My friend Barry Lynch, Sean Fleming's former bass player, had completed a master's degree in Media Ecology at New York University (NYU) a few years earlier. When Barry played with Sean, we talked endlessly about the courses he was taking. In particular, Barry talked about one of his professors, Neil Postman, as if he were a guru.

I went down to NYU in lower Manhattan on a summer afternoon with the intention of getting some information on their various master's programs, including Media Ecology. I went into the communications building I heard Barry talk about so often and met with a professor in his mid 60s. He answered my questions about the program but quickly changed the subject and asked me all kinds of questions about Ireland and my music career. People were coming and going, and he had a gentle and often hilarious banter with them. He made time for everyone be it the mail person, the cleaning staff or another professor in the department.

I was surprised he was listening intently to what I had to say. I was a rock-and-roll guitar player and didn't exactly consider myself an intellectual. I looked at my watch at one point and realized we had been talking for well over two hours. I asked him what I needed to do to get into the Media Ecology program. He said with a wry smile on his face, "Seamus, you're already in. Welcome to New York University." It turned out it was Neil Postman, the famous author and chairman of the Media Ecology program, I was talking to all that time. I nearly died of embarrassment. That started an unlikely friendship that lasted until his death in 2003. Fleming's and Ginny had awakened me from my physical and emotional sleep. Over the next several years, Postman and his band of gypsies would awaken me from my intellectual sleep.

In the fall of 1987, I attended my first lecture at NYU. While I had learned to read during my college experience, I was in no way prepared for the level of scholarship that awaited me at NYU. The media program was really a study of some of the great anthropology books of our time. It traced the development of communications from the hieroglyphics on the walls of ancient Egyptian caves all the way up to cable TV which was taking hold in the mid-80s.

The program was based on the foundational teachings of Marshall McLuhan, the Canadian semantics theorist who coined the term "The Medium is the Message." Postman studied under McLuhan and they lectured together extensively. He was seen as the interpreter of McLuhan's often complex and confusing ideas. Thanks to Postman and his colleagues, I developed the ability to look a lot deeper into the whole communications process, in particular the media. I always had a fascination with news broadcasting but studying with Postman and his colleagues gave me the tools to look at media—and indeed life—through a different lens. Like my early college day at Montclair, I could almost feel my brain evolving and opening up by the day. I questioned everything I thought I knew from religion, the media and history, to my own personal beliefs and the way I experienced life. It was a true metamorphosis—completely life altering. I enjoyed sharing all my new knowledge with Ginny. She was a great sounding board for all the new ideas swirling around in my head and well capable of challenging me at every turn.

I had the great fortune to meet an incredible mix of fellow students at NYU. There was Kierstan from Germany, two girls from Greece, another from Korea, a few from China and students from all over the U.S. The Media Ecology department had a wonderful culture. There were many days I walked by Postman's desk and ended up chatting for hours just like our first meeting. He was masterful at asking probing and provocative questions, triggering parts of my brain that had never been used before. He had a tremendous Jewish sense of humor and an ability to take the most complex material and turn it into plain English that even I could understand.

During those long afternoons, we were joined by several other students and professors, often getting into heated arguments about the political events of the day or the latest book we had read. We argued about ideas over many cups of coffee and my thoughts were treated with the same gravitas as the rest of the group. It was a far cry from St. Enda's where I was constantly told "dun do chlab," meaning "shut your mouth."

As part of my studies at NYU, I took summer courses in Holland, Germany and Ireland. During those intense week-long sessions, we were immersed in the culture of each country and worked closely with the host country's universities. The academics wanted to impress Postman and his young proteges. We often had raucous three-hour sessions discussing how the media was impacting the political landscape globally or how we were being dumbed down because television news had become "infotainment." Those were radical ideas at the time. The discussions spilled over to the bars and restaurants where we gathered late into the night and early morning, challenging each other's though process and stretching our brains as the drink loosened our tongues.

In Germany, just a few months before the fall of the Berlin Wall, we had a week-long course titled, "The Book." We stayed in Mainz, home of the Gutenberg Museum and the site of the first printing press where the Gutenberg Bible was published in the 1450s. Postman had a reverential love of the written word. On the day we toured the museum, I could see the emotion in his eyes as the curator showed us one of the first printings of the Gutenberg Bible. Postman and I got along great and he was always ready to engage in conversation, but I remember distinctly leaving him alone for a while as we left the museum. It was clear to me from his body language he needed time to process the deep emotions he was experiencing. I'm sure what he was feeling was something similar to what I felt that day back in 1974 when I walked into Manny's Music in New York. For me, that was my holy ground; for Postman, it was the Guttenberg Museum in Mainz.

Postman was quite famous in Germany, so we got the VIP treatment everywhere we went. We had full access to major museums and closed-book collections across the country. In one particular library, our group was looking at a collection of books and handwritten letters from Martin Luther. The letters were read out loud by a student in the group who happened to be a scholar on Luther and the Reformation. It was a surreal moment for all of us. Those letters had changed the course of history and we were able to touch them and pass them around.

When I asked the curator if he had any old music manuscripts, he took me into a dusty room and produced one of the oldest examples of written music tablature. The rest of the group followed. They said afterwards the look on my face when I saw the music tablature was priceless. It was like I had seen a ghost. Music is at the very core of my being—I think of it every hour of every day. Seeing one of the earliest pieces of music was truly a spiritual experience.

Taking those trips to Europe, often with the same people, allowed me to develop some wonderful friendships. As hectic as the courses were, there was plenty of time to get to know people socially. It was also an opportunity to wallow in my newfound ability to engage with people intellectually and expand my horizons.

During all this time, Ginny and I were still dating. She got a job at Montefiore Hospital in the Bronx working in epidemiology, her area of specialty. At that point, we should have been focused on our long-term plans, but I was holding onto my single life. I was afraid to let go of it by making a long-term commitment and that put a strain on our relationship.

Heartstrings

For my graduation from NYU, I had to do a thesis or a project. The thesis didn't appeal to me, so I suggested to the department chairman, Terry Moran, that I make a documentary on the role of music in film. Moran was former military and took zero bullshit from anyone. But he had a great mind and a deep love of music. In another environment, the chairman might have said, "That's not going to work." But Moran said, "Kelleher, you have to learn the craft. Take a course in filmmaking and write up your proposal." I took a four-month film course, did long hours of research and submitted the proposal to Moran. After getting his blessing, I went about making my film Heartstrings.

It was from my involvement with Ronan Downs and our charity organization Celtic Care that I got my idea for the documentary. I interviewed six homeless ladies living at a Red Cross shelter near Times Square. I interspersed those interviews with stereotypical comments about the homeless from regular people on the streets. It never ceases to amaze me what people are willing to say or do on camera. I also interviewed some of the staff of the American Red Cross. The documentary was supposed to be five minutes long but ended up being half an hour. It was paid for by some friends who owed me favors because of music I had done for them when they made low-budget films.

As part of my graduation requirements for the master's degree, I had to present my project to the faculty in the Media Ecology department. I rented a big room in the student center at NYU and had two giant TV screens set up. Also, I hired a catering service for a reception after my presentation. I rented a tux for the evening and sent formal invitations to my fellow students and the faculty from the Media Department. I invited the ladies whom I interviewed for the film along with the administrative staff from the Red Cross. The room was full. The lights went dark and I hit the start button on the VCR. The next half an hour was one of the most moving experiences I've ever had. The homeless ladies, watching their stories unfold on two big screens for the first time began to cry as did many in the audience. I wondered if they felt exploited or if they saw what I saw: six incredibly brave women. I had written "Heartstrings," the theme music for the film. As soon as the film ended, I got back on stage and performed the soundtrack live. My idea was to see what emotions the music would evoke without the screen images. It was an experiment with no right or wrong answer.

I thanked the homeless ladies for sharing their intimate stories and the Red Cross for letting me make the film. I also thanked Terry Moran for allowing me to do something completely different from what others were doing for graduation. The film was funded by Tim and Michael Kramer, two dear friends who had placed enormous trust in me.

The homeless women were fully engaged with the audience members and the NYU faculty during the reception. They were dressed up in their finery as if going out on the town. Each of them thanked me for giving them an opportunity and a forum to tell their personal story. I knew there was a minibus waiting outside the theatre to take them back to the confines and safety of the Red Cross shelter. I admired those individuals for their bravery in the face of all kinds of adversity. As I watched them depart NYU, I wondered where they would end up. But at least for one evening, I was able to shine the light on what they were going through.

As the reception ended, Terry Moran said, "Kelleher, that's how it's done. I only wish the other students would put that kind of effort and professionalism into their final presentations." Coming from Moran, that was the equivalent of an Academy Award.

California Dreaming

In January of 1989, I toured the West Coast of America with Sean Fleming. We had gigs in Las Vegas and Los Angeles. I flew into Las Vegas, and after our shows were finished, I rented a car and drove to LA, taking advantage of the opportunity to see another part of the country. Driving through the desert was an exhilarating experience. I was enthralled by its expanse and the constantly changing landscape. One minute, it was pure desert with cactus plants of all shapes and sizes protruding from the parched earth. Then, there were hundreds of wind turbines glistening on top of the hills like propellers on huge airplanes about to take off. Oil wells dotted the landscape like ants bobbing up and down on a bed of sand. I played the music of Eric Clapton, Rory Gallagher, Jimi Hendrix and B.B. King loudly on the car stereo. My spirits were buoyed by the clear blue skies, the beaming sun and the broad spectacular vistas that went on forever.

My sister Maura asked me to visit some friend of hers in Burbank when I got to LA. I had come out of my shell in the safe confines of Fleming's and New York but socializing with strangers didn't appeal to me. After Maura mentioned my upcoming trip to California, her friend Marge called to invite me to dinner in their home in Burbank. I agreed to a short visit. After arriving in LA, I knocked on the door of Joe and Marge Shields' home and was welcomed into the house by their daughters Mary Pat and Colleen. They weren't just good looking; they were absolutely beautiful.

This was too good to be true. I knew I wasn't going anywhere after an hour if I could help it. I felt like calling my sister Maura to thank her. Joe and Marge were great company as were their daughters. We talked for hours about every subject under the sun and they insisted I stay the night. The two girls took me out to some local bars in Burbank to meet their friends. We hit it off right away and talked and laughed all night long. Both girls had a great sense of humor, a quality I value in any friendship.

The next day, I was to move to an apartment available to the band as part of our weekend booking in Des Reagan's, a well-established bar in Burbank. Joe and Marge said they would love to have me stay at their home. Despite their hospitality and the fun I had with Colleen and Mary Pat, I didn't want to impose on them.

Chris Ebneth had replaced Chris Bishop in the Sean Fleming Band— Bishop wanted to focus on his solo career. Chris Ebneth had a long history with Sean, so the transition from one Chris to another was seamless. We went into the band apartment atop Des Reagan's and, because it was in rough shape, decided we couldn't stay there, despite it being free accommodation. We found a small motel close by but it felt seedy and they were charging an arm and a leg for our week-long stay. Just as I was about to book the room, I decided to call the Shields to see if their offer to stay was still open. I told them I had my buddy Chris from the band with me. Without a moment's hesitation, they said to come right over.

We stayed with the Shields for a week. The family came to see the band at Des Reagan's and, by strange coincidence, Colleen was working there as a waitress. I spent a lot of time with Mary Pat and Colleen over the week just hanging out. I also got to know Joe and Marge very well. Chris and I toured around Los Angeles and went to San Diego for a few days to see the zoo and SeaWorld. By the time I left the Shields' home to head back to New York, I had taken a shine to Mary Pat. She was twenty-one and in her third year of college and I was in my thirties. The chances of her showing any interest in me seemed out of the question but there was "something about Mary."

A Day Like No Other

I awoke on May 15, 1989, my graduation day from NYU, with an anticipation I could almost touch. The graduation ceremony took place in Washington Square Park, the epicenter of the NYU campus. Ginny was with me as was Chris Bishop, my good friend from the Sean Fleming Band. Decked out in my cap and gown, I made my way from the department building over to the park pondering the two amazing years I spent on campus in the heart of the city I loved so much.

As I entered the park, the Emerald Police Pipe Band played "Amazing Grace." That was all I needed—much like the time I entered the stadium at Montclair State College and saw my Dad five years earlier—tears welled up in my eyes. I wondered what Dad and Mam would think of their son, who showed no interest in college after high school, receiving a master's degree from one of the world's most prestigious universities.

I took my seat with the thousands of other graduates as trumpeters let loose with "Pomp and Circumstance" from the top of the majestic Washington Square Arch. Rituals are important to me—they mark time—and they mark accomplishment. I was proud of the work I had done at NYU. I had learned a lot academically and graduated near the top of my class. I learned how to make a documentary and I gained the respect of some of the great minds at the school. I could engage with people in possession of intellects far superior to mine. Probably my biggest takeaway was that I learned to always look at the other side of an argument. I often refer to that as embracing the art of the dialectic. By doing so, you can understand the world around you and learn to respect others who may have differing opinions to yours. I had no idea what I was going to do with my newfound knowledge, but on May 15, 1989, it didn't matter. It was a time to celebrate.

After graduation, I had lunch with Ginny and we met up with Terry Moran in McSorley's bar for a few drinks. McSorley's is one of the oldest bars in New York, dating back to 1854, and renowned for the sawdust on the floor and a policy of not letting women drink at the bar, although that had changed many years earlier. The owner of McSorley's, Matty Maher, a good friend of Terry and a colorful character full of life, regaled us with story after story.

During that afternoon at the pub, Terry asked me about my future plans. I told him I would love to continue my graduate studies but felt that intellectually, I was not at that level. "Kelleher, you are," he said in his normal, short, no-bullshit style. Within a few months, I had taken the various exams and was accepted into the PhD program at NYU. Just the very idea was daunting, especially being surrounded by the likes of Postman, Moran and their group of towering intellectuals. I'm still not sure why they had adopted me, but there I was in the middle of it all. On several occasions, they had me sit in on interviews for incoming PhD candidates. I had come a long way from my first day at Montclair State where I could barely read the syllabus and had to rely on those Cliff Notes. The work was very difficult at the PhD level, but I still enjoyed it and was able to keep up most of the time.

Ginny and I stayed together for well over a year after graduation. I'm not exactly sure how or why Ginny and I drifted apart, but I know my lack of willingness to make a long-term commitment and my alcohol intake were a big part of it. I was drinking way too much, and I wasn't at my best when alcohol was involved.

On the surface, life looked like it was going great for me. I was with a rocking band, had just finished my master's degree, and was working on a PhD, but there was a dark side.

I was blacking out on a regular basis after drinking. I woke many mornings trying to reconstruct what had happened the night before. I hated who I was on those mornings. I squandered many opportunities that came my way both musically and academically. Because Ginny lived in the Bronx and I was still in Manhattan, I was able to hide much of my drinking life from her. I didn't want the party to end.

Eventually, Ginny moved to Baltimore to continue her work in epidemiology. We stayed friends and she came to see me perform with the Sean Fleming Band when we played in Washington. She played a major role in helping me discover who I really was, and I'll never forget her for that. She was from a lovely family who always made me feel welcome in their home. Had we met at another time in my life, things may have been different between us.

Warning Signs

While the heady days of MTV were behind us, the Sean Fleming Band was as popular as ever. Fleming's was still crowded on weekends and, amazingly, there were only a few changes in the staff. We were like family and it was hard for anyone to leave.

We had a Mexican bus boy at Fleming's named Refugio. I was very close with him. He was one of the hardest workers I have ever seen, always with a big smile on his face. The staff and all the customers loved him. He became part of our family and part of our many social gatherings outside work.

We noticed after a while that Refugio was drinking an awful lot. We all tried to help him, but he continued to drink and do drugs, making it impossible for him to hold a job. He was eventually hospitalized suffering from HIV and his entire body shut down. My friend Ronan and I visited him, as did many of the staff from Fleming's. We watched this beautiful human being wither away in front of our eyes. He died at the tender age of 20.

Watching my friend Refugio's decline unfold should have been a clear sign to me that my own drinking was out of hand, but I continued with my self-destructive behavior. Night after night I was drinking more than ever before. I let myself and my bandmates down on stage by not being able to perform at my best. For the most part, I managed to avoid the scourge of drugs, but alcohol was my drug of choice and despite all the indications, I wouldn't admit I had a problem.

After Ginny moved to Baltimore, I spent a lot of time with Ella O'Sullivan, my friend of many years who worked for Aer Lingus. Initially, we just met for drinks but after a few months, romance entered the picture. We kissed one night as she was getting in a taxi back to her apartment in Queens. I don't think either of us were expecting that one short kiss to turn our long friendship into a romance.

Ella had a great personality and loved being out with friends. She could drink ten Irish coffees and still walk a straight line. I, on the other hand, was not in control of my drinking. Within a short while, we were out drinking several nights a week. I then did the most stupid thing I ever did by lighting a cigarette for myself at age 38. I was out with Ella and some friends and lit up for a joke more than anything else. I knew cigarettes played a big role in my mother's ill health and contributed to her passing at such an early age. Within a very short period I was hooked, and it was unusual to find me at the bar without a Parliament cigarette in one hand and a Jameson whiskey in the other.

From 1987 to 2014, my life could be categorized by what I was drinking at the time. The Dom Pérignon Period: 1987-1988. The Tequila Period: 1988-1992. The Brandy Period: 1988-1990. The Irish Mist Period: 1990-1995. The Red Wine Period: 1995-2000. The Jameson or Golden Era: 2000-2014. Clearly, those periods often overlapped as I rarely refused any hard liquor that came my way, but there were certain personality traits that came out during each period. The Dom Pérignon was the happy Seamus. It was my first time getting a real buzz on and things rarely got out of control. The Tequila Period was characterized by a more aggressive Seamus. The shyness was gone, and I developed a sort of swagger on and off stage. I talked to everyone and was ready to join in on any activity. I also experienced an awakening of my sexuality with tequila. I knew the ladies enjoyed the guitar playing and, in a strange sense, I felt I was teasing them when I walked on top of the bar in Fleming's holding the bottle of tequila to my lips. Remember, I was skinny, had that rocking mullet hairdo, wore tight-fitting leather pants and was playing guitar with my teeth in one of the hottest spots in New York. It was a perfect storm.

The brandy phase could be broken into sub-sections. First came Rémy Martin VSOP, then Hennessy and then anything with VSOP on it. The highlight of the Brandy Period was at a house party gig in New Jersey with Gerry, the same guy who used to buy Dom Pérignon for the band at Fleming's. Gerry's wife mistakenly gave me an oversized Waterford Crystal tumbler of Louis XIII instead of regular brandy. Instantly, I knew this drink was different. I was like Pooh bear with the honey, I savored every last drop. Eventually, Gerry handed me the bottle and said, "Seamus, I can't think of anyone who deserves this more." The Louis XIII bottle was Baccarat Crystal and cost over $200—and that's without the brandy.

I always associate my Irish Mist Period with Eamonn Doran's and the Green Derby. How many nights did I sit at the bar at Eamonn's with my Parliament cigarettes and a huge snifter with the thick Irish Mist creating ever-moving patterns along the side of the glass? The drink was appropriately named as I missed a lot because of the it. I often had no clue how I made it home.

By the early nineties, I continued to wake up many mornings in a haze. Sometimes, I had no memory at all, which scared me, but not enough to make me stop.

There were prostitutes on the streets surrounding Fleming's. They had been moved up from Times Square when the Mayor of New York, Ed Koch, was attempting to clean up the area. One night, after being over-served in Fleming's, I left to walk the five blocks home. The staff at

Fleming's didn't realize how drunk I was. I staggered into walls and doorways when one of the ladies of the night said, "Mr. Guitar Man, you need to go back to your friends at the bar." My good Samaritan and her friend took me by the arm and walked me back to Fleming's where she told the doorman he needed to get me home safe. The lady never asked for anything in return for her kind deed. She was used to seeing me walk home most nights where I wasn't wall banging. She knew there was something wrong, even if I didn't.

One thing I did not do on a regular basis were drugs, and I believe that is the only reason I'm still here and able to share my story. Drugs were rampant all over New York during the 1980s and '90s. Despite my drinking and the changes that were occurring in my life, I was naïve in many ways. I was oblivious to the fact that most people around me were doing cocaine. I tried it a few times with some musician friends and loved it. Cocaine made me feel confident and invincible. I was stunned one morning when a news headline splashed across the TV screen saying Len Bias, a superstar basketball player and one of my favorite athletes, died from a heart attack brought on by an overdose of cocaine. I did cocaine once more after that and my heart started racing as the image of Len Bias went through my head. That was enough to scare me. I never touched cocaine again.

Ella was very popular and well respected within the Irish business community. She introduced me to some great people. For the first time since I had come to America, I began attending Irish community events in New York. Celtic Care, the charity organization I cofounded with Ronan, was doing very well. Our boat ride on the Circle Line each summer was the highlight of the year for many in the Irish community. Ella was a big supporter of what I was doing and often did the heavy lifting for us. I had two other dear friends, Martha and Helaine from the financial services world, who also helped raise a huge amount of money for the homeless.

The First Friday

After I got my master's degree, Terry Moran asked me to join him and some friends for lunch on the first Friday of every month, which I started attending in 1990. It was at Eamonn Doran's and included Frank McCourt, his brother Malachy and a cast of characters ranging from the Irish Ambassador to the UN and the Irish Consul General of New York, to people like Mary Higgins Clark. Frank McCourt had retired from teaching at Stuyvesant High School a few years earlier. His brother, Malachy, was the raucous McCourt one during our lunch meetings. Often, ten or fifteen of us would be sitting in Doran's and, without warning, Malachy would stand up and come out with some bizarre rant to the entire restaurant. I was shocked at first but after a few months I got used to it. Malachy was a regular Broadway performer and was also featured in numerous films and TV shows. Eamonn Doran's was just another stage for his wonderful talents.

I was the young kid on the block during those lunches and everyone was incredibly welcoming, especially the McCourt brothers, who made sure I was introduced to everyone in the room. Within a few years, Frank McCourt's Angela's Ashes shot to fame. After that, the First Friday meetings became a forum for posers trying to be seen with the McCourt brothers. I felt privileged to know the brothers and the First Friday crew before things changed.

A Dream Job

In late 1991, I got a phone call from a friend asking if I would be interested in auditioning for an Irish TV show that had just started in New York. They needed someone to do interviews. I'm not sure how they heard of me. I took the subway to Brooklyn, where New York City's public television station was located. It was an amazing facility with multiple studios. I always had a fascination with the whole production side of television. After an hour watching several people audition for the role of host, it was my turn. There were three cameras and a big stage. For the audition, I had to interview some musicians. That was helpful, as I knew them from the various festivals where we shared a stage. As nervous as I was, once the camera started rolling, I felt a strange sense of calm and enjoyed every second of it. The producer asked me to stay where I was after the first interview and sent out several other interviewees for me to talk to. Some of the people I didn't know, but I just kept asking them questions and it all seemed so natural.

I got a call the next day asking if I could come back the following week to do more interviews. I was now officially part of Erin's Focus, an Irish TV show that aired in New York every Saturday between 5-5:30 pm on Channel 3, a cable station. The production company had a second show Irish Eyes where I also did interviews. This was the era where there were just a few cable stations to choose from. Channel 3 was wedged between CBS (Channel 2) and NBC (Channel 4). A lot of New Yorkers flicked through the channels watching sports on Saturday afternoons and stumbled on Erin's Focus in the process.

Within a short time, people in Fleming's were coming up to me saying they saw me on TV. It was good for my ego. On any given Saturday, I was interviewing a well-known sports figure, a politician or a musician. The staff at the studio were great. I shared hosting duties with Anne Tarrant, a beautiful and super-talented lady also from Ireland.

I had a great critic whom I met most Saturday nights at Doran's. Joe Ruane was a New York legend. He had been a bartender, a promoter and an entrepreneur. Like Eamonn Doran, he had helped hundreds of young Irish get a start in New York. He was involved with promoting the top Irish artists of the day. He watched Erin's Focus and Irish Eyes each week and gave me an honest blow-by-blow critique. He was a big fan of what I was doing and saw a bright future for me in television.

Despite my drinking, I was on top of my game. The band was going great, I was doing well at NYU and I was fast becoming a TV personality. And then it got even better.

In the spring of 1992. I got a call from Niall O'Dowd, the editor and publisher of the *Irish Voice* newspaper in New York, telling me that I had been voted Community Person of the Year, in a write-in ballot in his paper. The award was being given jointly by the newspaper and Aer Lingus, the Irish national airline. The *Voice* was one of only a few major Irish newspapers in the U.S. so it was a big deal. I was humbled by such an honor.

Speaking the Truth

A week after I found out about the Community Person of the Year award, Ella took me to meet some friends for brunch at the Old Stand bar on Third Ave. I was hung over after being in Doran's till 5 am that morning and did everything to get out of the brunch date but to no avail. I walked in the door only to be met by almost a hundred people. I looked around to see what folks were celebrating when they yelled "surprise" and started to congratulate me on being named Community Person of the Year. I was totally caught off guard. I didn't know what to do.

Ella did a great job gathering co-workers from Fleming's, fellow students and faculty at NYU, and my colleagues in the television world. It sunk in that the award was real and it was special. My professors at NYU were proud of their Irish offspring, even though I'm sure they saw me as a bit of an oddball between my music, my love of academics and my new-found television fame.

A day that started off on such a high note went downhill fast. As the afternoon progressed, I got increasingly belligerent and rude. Sitting at the bar in the Old Stand, Ella said, "Seamus, I think you might be an alcoholic." She was not being nasty even though she had reason to be, but she saw something in me after that day's drinking she didn't like. I was shocked to hear those words from her—she was a straight shooter—I was mad. I couldn't look her in the eye and left the bar abruptly on my own. It wasn't that I got violent or crazy when I drank to excess, it was more a loss of my dignity and, along with it, the good side of Seamus. Ella was right, I was indeed an alcoholic but not ready to admit it. She was speaking the truth.

The Plaza Surprise

Ella and I patched things up after a few days, and I promised to be more careful with the drink. The Community Awards ceremony took place at the Plaza Hotel in New York. Before the actual ceremony, I did an interview in Gaelic with Sean Ban Breathnach, one of Ireland's best-known broadcasters. It was interesting to say the least as I speak very little Gaelic. It was broadcast a few days later much to the amusement of my brothers-in-law, who are fluent Gaelic speakers. I was also interviewed by a reporter from The *Connaught Tribune*, the main newspaper in my hometown of Galway.

Before I got to the Plaza for the actual awards ceremony, I got the surprise of my life when my sisters Geraldine and Carol arrived from Ireland courtesy of Aer Lingus. I'm sure Ella had something to do with that. I was speechless. So much was happening all at once. I was on a high. Now I could share this special day with my immediate family. My Aunt Nora was also there. She was in her element since like me, she had a love affair with New York City and the Plaza was its epicenter.

As the awards were handed out, I looked around the beautiful ornate and opulent room and saw the faces of people who I had come to know well in my 18 years in New York: some from my music, some from NYU and random people I met on my long, crazy journey. My only disappointment was that Ronan Downs, the cofounder of Celtic Care, wasn't also on the stage that night. He was the inspiration for the work I did with the homeless.

So here I was with all this attention. It lasted a bit longer than the proverbial fifteen minutes, but there was trouble on the horizon. I received a letter in the mail from a good friend with a newspaper clipping regarding the producer of Erin's Focus. There was concern regarding some shady finances. This quickly became public knowledge in the close-knit Irish community in New York. Receiving the Community Person of the Year award and the attention it afforded put me in an awkward situation. In my role of co-founder and leader of Celtic Care, I knew I could not be associated with Erin's Focus as long as the producer stayed there. After a late-night conversation with Niall O'Dowd and Jim Lyndon, the head of PR at Aer Lingus, I made a difficult decision to resign from Erin's Focus. It was a hard thing to do as I loved hosting the show. I was getting better every day on camera, the feedback from the TV audience was positive and guests specifically asked that I interview them. The opportunities seemed endless, but in the blink of an eye, it was over. Although I tried, I never had the same opportunity to get back on air even with the support of the *Irish Voice*, Aer Lingus and other movers and shakers in the Irish community.

Meanwhile back in Los Angeles

Since meeting Mary Pat in 1989, we continued to talk on the phone every few months purely as friends. Our conversations covered many topics. Her degree was in communications, so sometimes we talked about the media and how it impacted our lives. We were both in relationships and exchanged war stories about our ups and downs. I remember many times saying half-jokingly, "Mary Pat, why don't we just get married; we could avoid all the drama?" It was always met with a holler of laughter, which confirmed to me that it would never happen.

In the early '90s, I planned a trip to California just so I would have an excuse to meet up with Mary Pat again in person. Her parents knew by then I wanted to be more than just friends. To my utter dismay, I only saw Mary Pat for about five minutes before she got in a car with her boyfriend and headed back to college in San Diego. It was stupid of me not to check her romantic status before I made the trip cross country, but regardless, I was utterly deflated and felt embarrassed after making such an idiot of myself. I refer to that as "The California Massacre." It was the first of many. I immediately went to the nearest travel agent and booked a week-long trip to Acapulco, Mexico. I sat on the beach for several days wondering how I could be such a fool to think I could convince someone like Mary Pat to take a romantic liking to me.

In 1991, Mary Pat was selected as the Los Angeles representative for the Rose of Tralee festival in Ireland. It's an annual event held in Ireland where cities from the Irish diaspora all over the world choose a girl, or "Rose," to represent them in the festival. It's not your typical beauty pageant. While good looks play a role, and Mary Pat was beautiful, it's all about the personalities of the contestants and their ability to impress the judges over the course of the week-long festival. Mary Pat being selected as the Los Angeles Rose was a big deal with all kinds of media coverage in Los Angeles and in Ireland.

Mary Pat stopped by New York on her way to the festival and stayed at my apartment on the Upper East Side for a few days. I had known her now for a few years and had deep feelings for her. Despite my numerous failed attempts to woo her, I tried everything to impress her during the New York trip to get something going on the romantic front. I took her to all the hot spots in the city, but she was having none of it. Her body language made it clear we were mere friends. If I tried to bring the subject around to a potential relationship, the conversation went silent. I tried a walk through Central Park as that always worked before with the ladies, but not with Mary Pat. Next on the list was the Circle Line where I did my best Leonardo DiCaprio, but as soon as I tried to hold hands, she put them deep in her pockets.

Finally, I took her to Eamonn Doran's. I figured that was my ace in the hole since I was a mini celebrity there. Our visit was carefully choreographed. I made sure to let my favorite waitress know I was on a mission. She fussed over us both and we were ushered to the best table in the house. Eamonn himself came over to say hello. Drinks were being sent over to us by everyone. Sean the bartender also knew about the mission and did everything to help me win Mary Pat over. I said hello to the hugely popular film producer Jim Sheridan and he said "Hello Seamus" back. With all due respect to Mr. Sheridan, Mary Pat didn't even notice; in fact, she was anxious to get home to read her book.

The following evening, Mary Pat went to dinner with an old college friend, and I went out with Ella whom I was still seeing from time to time.

When I came back to the apartment, my tongue loosened by a few drinks, I professed my love for Mary Pat saying, "I adore you and I'll never marry again unless I love someone as much as I love you." She didn't call me a blithering fool, but she didn't have to. She said, "I'm very flattered but I have a boyfriend." I knew I crossed a red line and figured I had ruined any chance of us getting together. That was one long, awkward night. It was the Upper East Side Massacre. Mary Pat got on a plane to Ireland the next day, glad to be rid of this very persistent and annoying Galway man.

The Boston Massacre

Fast forward two years, and Mary Pat's was visiting her sister Colleen in Boston who was preparing for the birth of her second child. I got wind of this and decided to give it one last shot. When I want something, I tend to be tenacious and lose all sense of reality and common sense.

I had just gotten an old Volkswagen GT from my friend Chris Ebneth. It was a great little car, but the driver's side had a hole in front of the brake pedal that got bigger by the day, and one of the wipers didn't work. It was also a stick shift, and I had never driven one before. But the mixture of love and stupidity knows no boundaries, so I said, "Screw it, I'm going to Boston."

I set off on what should have been a four-hour journey. The weather was horrific and I had my hand out the window most of the drive trying to clear the windshield. Cold water came up from the highway through the hole in the floor soaking my clothes. I'm sure I was in third gear for a good portion of the trip as changing gears was risking life and limb, especially in the bad weather. I didn't stop the car for fear of it not starting again.

I arrived in Boston after a harrowing five-and-a-half-hour drive. I was met at Colleen's apartment door by Mary Pat. She was as radiant as ever with that smile I loved so much. I made believe I had some work to do in Boston and thought it would be nice to just pop in and say hello. After a few hours, I asked Mary Pat out to dinner. Colleen stayed home and we found a restaurant close by in case she went into labor. We had a nice time, but it was not exactly the romantic interlude I hoped for. I tried all my best lines and moves, but as in my previous attempts, it was a dismal failure. In desperation, I tried to give her a kiss as I left Colleen's apartment that evening, but my sad attempt barely grazed the side of her cheek. I tried again and grazed the other cheek as she turned her head for a second time. I was mortified. The Boston Massacre was just one more hit to my ego.

I was used to being the center of attention in Fleming's and didn't have to work that hard connecting with girls. But the one girl I wanted showed no interest in me whatsoever. I drove through the streets of Boston in torrential rain in search of a hotel. I booked into a Holiday Inn and sat at a tacky karaoke bar for two hours listening to Bostonians singing horrible music while I drained several glasses of wine and chain-smoked Parliament cigarettes. A few weeks after the debacle in Boston, Colleen's baby, Ryan, was born. Mary Pat made her way back to Seattle where she worked at a family camp in the mountains. I was done chasing her— maybe.

I went back to Ireland on vacation that summer. I knew that Fleming's was coming to an end. The Sean Fleming Band had played there since the night it opened in 1982. A twelve-year residency was a rare thing in New York. The actual bar was now run down since little money had been reinvested in it over the years, and the lease was up. It was still crowded at weekends, but the end was near.

For the first time in many years, I lost my passion for the music. It was real work and my guitar playing was stagnant. It had been a great ride with Sean, but he was such a strong front man, it was hard for me to establish an identity of my own. Much like my trip to Spain in 1979, the trip back home to Ireland was an attempt to figure out my next move.

Victory at Last

My visit home ended up being something special. I spent a lot of time with my sisters and I reconnected with many friends around Galway. My sisters and I are best friends. I can talk to them about anything, so they were a great sounding board for me as I tried to figure things out. They knew all about the saga with Mary Pat.

As it turned out, Mary Pat and her parents were visiting my sister Maura. I only found that out when I arrived in Ireland. I stayed with my sister Carol just down the street from Maura. I had zero interest in another massacre with Mary Pat, especially in my hometown. I had given it my best shot in Boston, almost killing myself on interstate 95 in the process a few months earlier.

I met a great musician friend, Kevin Garvey, in town and he asked me to join him for a session later that evening in a little bar called Myles Lee. The "session" is an Irish tradition where musicians come together and play music in an informal setting. Everyone is welcome to participate. My sister Carol suggested I call Mary Pat to see if she wanted to go into town with me. Reluctantly, I called her, without any thought other than for her to enjoy the session at Myles Lee. To my surprise she said she would love to go.

On the way into town, we stopped off at Trigger Martin's for a quiet drink before meeting up with my musician friends. Ironically, Trigger Martin's used to be the Genoa Bar where I worked as a bartender before leaving Ireland in 1975. We were only there for fifteen minutes but in that short time span, something changed between us. Maybe it was that I stopped trying so hard, or maybe it was that Mary Pat had been worked on by her parents, both of whom liked me. Regardless, we had a lovely time and then went across the street holding hands to Myles Lee.

The session kicked into gear when we got there. Kevin was a wonderful singer/songwriter and a fine guitarist. I pulled up a chair and took out my guitar. Kevin and I sang everything from Cat Stevens' "Wild World" and Thin Lizzy's "Whiskey in The Jar" to many traditional Irish songs. We were high on the music and oblivious to the large crowd that gathered. Mary Pat was having a blast and beaming. For the first time, she saw me in my own environment, where I was just focused on the music and my friends. I stopped trying to coerce her into liking me. I was just being me. It was a night etched in my memory forever. We continued to hold hands that evening after Myles Lee and when we had our first kiss, my heart was racing. Mercifully, another massacre had been averted in my hometown.

I woke up the next day and asked myself, "What happened last night?" I only had two drinks, so the magical images of Myles Lee and Trigger Martin's were clear in my head. Later that day, Mary Pat, her mom and dad and I gathered in Maura's house to watch the annual Rose of Tralee pageant that Mary Pat had participated in just a few years earlier. At the end of the evening, we sat on the steps of Maura's apartment talking into the early hours. I had several drinks and summoned up the courage to ask Mary Pat if she would ever consider having a long-term relationship with me. "Do you think, maybe, perhaps…?" To my utter disbelief, she said "yes." I didn't know what to say. I was stunned.

The following day, I had to leave for Shannon Airport to get back to New York for a gig. Mary Pat was staying in Ireland for another week, and we agreed to talk when she got back to America. I arrived at Shannon only to find my flight was delayed for six or seven hours. I called Mary Pat just to say hello and suggested she come down to hang out. She agreed. I was over the moon. She left for Shannon, but within an hour, the flight for New York was called and I had to get on the plane knowing Mary Pat was on her way to see me.

I panicked and felt my skin crawl. I didn't know what to do. The gig in New York was a wedding and had been booked for over a year. I couldn't let the bride and groom down as they were longtime friends. There were no cell phones to explain the situation to Mary Pat. I got on the plane an emotional mess. I finally made an impression on the woman I loved but I feared I might have blown it. I dealt with the situation the only way I knew how. I had a few glasses of red wine and many Jameson whiskies to wash away my sorrows.

The next few days were hard. All I could think of was Mary Pat. We did finally talk on the phone, and she was understanding about what transpired. Maybe she felt guilty for all the rejections and massacres she put me through.

A week later, Mary Pat had a stop-over in New York on her way back to Seattle. I met her at Kennedy Airport with a dozen roses in hand, not knowing what to expect. I thought she was just passing through, but she had changed her flight to allow for a 24-hour layover before her flight back West.

I was so relieved when she responded to my embrace and my kiss. My entire body was tingling. We went back to my railroad apartment on 83rd Street—the same one where I had made a fool of myself a few years earlier telling her I adored her. We stayed up talking most of the night. The next day, I drove her back to Kennedy Airport where she boarded a plane for Seattle. It was hard saying goodbye to her, but I knew something was finally brewing between us. There was hope, and I was prepared to do everything in my power to seize the moment.

We talked at least once or twice every day for the following two weeks with each conversation getting longer. I wanted to visit her right away to build on the momentum but couldn't get the time off as I was busy with the music. I decided it was time to make a bold move. Love knows no bounds with Seamus Kelleher. "I can't make it out there this weekend as I was hoping, but why don't I come to Seattle in two weeks' time and bring you back to New York with me?" That's exactly what I said to Mary Pat on the phone. I expected to hear howls of laughter but she didn't laugh. There was silence for what seemed like an eternity. I wondered if I had finally blown it, but then she said, "Ok, but this is not a dress rehearsal." Even back then, I knew that when Mary Pat said something, she meant it. Now in total shock, I mumbled, "What about I fly out to Seattle a week from next Saturday?" to which she replied, "That sounds good."

The next week was a whirlwind. I was afraid Mary Pat would change her mind. I was performing in Washington, DC that week with Sean Fleming and everything became one big jumble in my head. My way of life was about to change dramatically. For the first time in ten years, I was going to be living with a girl. Not just that, but there was every possibility this girl would become my wife. As Mary Pat made abundantly clear on the phone: this was not a dress rehearsal.

I had to declutter my apartment in a hurry, making sure evidence of any previous relationships and rendezvous were removed. Ten years as a bachelor is a long time. I realized I had no money for the flight and the long drive back across country from Seattle. I reached out to Sean Fleming. When I told him my story, he started laughing but I could tell he was happy for me. Sean's generosity has no limits and within a day $2,000 was deposited in my Allied Irish Bank account in Manhattan.

A week later, immediately after a show with Sean in Princeton, New Jersey, I made my way to Newark Airport and got on a plane to Seattle. Mary Pat and I had never really had a proper date other than the session at Myles Lee in Galway. Yet we were getting in Mary Pat's tiny Honda Civic to spend at least eight days and nights together driving across America.

Mary Pat met me at the airport in Seattle early on a Sunday morning. We arrived at Camp Huston in Gold Bar, a summer camp and retreat center for children, adults and families, where Mary Pat worked in administration. It was a beautiful, idyllic setting with lush green fields, streams and wooden cabins throughout. The staff were welcoming and it was immediately clear they were very fond of Mary Pat. I'm sure they wondered, as many people did, what was this rocker musician doing with such a beautiful woman?

The next day we went sightseeing. We went atop the iconic Seattle Space Needle and visited the famed Pike Place Fish Market. It was easy to see why Seattle had become a mecca for the youth of America. It's a beautiful part of the world and they had Nirvana, amazing coffee shops and Microsoft. It was the cool place to be.

The highpoint of the day was a boat trip on Puget Sound and a beautiful afternoon spent exploring San Juan Island. We were on our first real date, but it was as if we had been together for years. What I loved about Mary Pat from day one she didn't need to be talking all the time. We walked for a long period without a word between us just enjoying the beauty of the island and the spectacular Puget Sound surrounding us on all sides. In many ways, Mary Pat reminded me of my friend Brendan Glynn. She was easy to be with.

The next morning, we packed up her Honda Civic. I could tell Mary Pat was sad leaving a place she had come to love. There were no tears; it was just the look on her face. Sometimes it's good to know when to say nothing. Once we got in the car, I promised I would take her back to Seattle one day.

The Long Dance

Within a few minutes we were on interstate 90 and, according to the map, we had 2,920 miles to go before we hit the George Washington Bridge into New York.

Every American should drive across our country at least once. It's the only way to appreciate the scale and diversity of this remarkable land, geographically and culturally. As we made our way out into the desert, just like the time I drove from Vegas to LA, I was taken by the changing colors and contours of the landscape beneath the ever-changing sky. The sun was shining brightly as we drove through Washington State. In the distance, we saw beautiful black horses on top of a large hill. As we got closer, we realized they were statues made of iron. We were looking at a beautiful art sculpture "Grandfather Cuts Loose the Ponies," also known as the Wild Horse Monument. We walked up the hill and were treated to an extraordinary view that stretched for miles and miles before us.

We got back in the car and drove through small towns, not very different from the ones I saw in the cowboy and western movies I watched as a kid growing up in Ireland. I wondered what it was really like to live there for the early settlers. It was hard to imagine a life where the only transport was by horse or wagon if you were doing well. The isolation of it all was hard to fathom.

We each brought along a bunch of cassette tapes for the trip. As I sifted through her collection, I was delighted to see we had many tapes in common. In particular, we were both fans of a Galway band The Stunning. Their music became the soundtrack for the trip. Our favorite song was

"Brewing up a Storm." There certainly was a storm brewing, but in the best possible sense of the word.

Because of our limited budget, we only had eight days for the long drive. We took turns driving and napping. We made great progress and finally reached our first stop in Missoula, Montana. We found a nice little motel to rest our weary heads. We looked at each other realizing we had already committed to a long-term relationship without ever really having spent a lot of time together. For the first time, we were now going to spend the night together as a couple. We did that and more in every state along our journey. We laughed and we sang and danced and romanced as we made our way across America the Beautiful.

Our first major stop was Yellowstone National Park. It was early October. I'm not poetic enough to do justice to the majesty of Yellowstone. We spent a full day there and our breath was taken away at every turn, from the Old Faithful geyser to the Sulphur Springs bubbling up from underneath the surface of the earth. At one point, we pulled into an empty parking area to take a short nap. It was not tourist season so the park was fairly empty. An hour later, we woke to a herd of buffalo grazing on the vegetation all around us. It was a spectacular and hauntingly beautiful sight.

We climbed a mountainside road and as the elevation increased, snow fell in waves covering the parched earth like a light white blanket. Down at the base of the mountain, it was still 60 degrees with the sun beaming down on the beautiful landscape dressed up in a kaleidoscope of fall colors. We drove in silence for miles inhaling it all. We stayed the night in a motel outside the park and continued on our journey the next morning.

Our next destination was Mount Rushmore. It was exhilarating to see the images of presidents Washington, Jefferson, Lincoln and Roosevelt carved into rock. The pictures and videos I'd seen didn't capture the grandeur and pure scale of it all.

We passed through the Badlands on to South Bend, Indiana, where we stopped to visit the University of Notre Dame. I have always enjoyed American college football and was a fan of the Fighting Irish. We walked around the fabled campus and made our way to the football stadium. In my head I could hear the Notre Dame fight song echoing through the eighty-thousand capacity stadium under the watchful eye of the iconic giant mural of Touchdown Jesus.

From there it was on through Ohio and Pennsylvania where the lush green trees were starting to transform themselves with the first blush of fall. It was when we saw the sign for the George Washington Bridge crossing from New Jersey to New York Mary Pat fully realized her life was about to change dramatically. It was like she had seen a ghost. She went totally silent and her face was ashen as she started biting her nails. My initial thought was to comfort her by saying she would love New York but as I did when we left Seattle, I decided she needed to figure out what was happening and my well-intentioned words of comfort would get in the way. We drove down towards Manhattan on the Major Deegan Expressway mostly silent.

We arrived at my apartment in the early evening. The eerie silence continued as we unpacked but within a short time, I could see Mary Pat breathe again. That night we went out for a few drinks at Etcetera, my local bar, to help ease the anxiety we were both feeling as we began life as a couple. We had a lovely time just sitting at the bar talking about all we had seen and experienced during our incredible trip across country. I also introduced Mary Pat to Ronan Downs, the owner of Etcetera and my partner with Celtic Care. Ronan had the welcome of the world for Mary Pat and immediately put her at ease.

My neighborhood on the Upper East Side was a hub of activity. There were little stores and restaurants mixed in with small apartments buildings. You felt safe walking around the block, no matter what time of day or night. It was three blocks from the East River and six blocks from Gracie Mansion where the mayor of New York Rudy Giuliani made his home. There was a beautiful path along the river where New Yorkers walked, jogged or sat in chairs people-watching or enjoying the sunshine.

By the time Mary Pat arrived in New York, I knew many of my neighbors on my block. There was a great character Lucille who kept everyone in line. God forbid if you dropped some trash on the street or put something in the garbage that could be of use to someone like a pair of shoes with plenty of wear left in them. Those items were carefully placed on the sidewalk for someone in need. Her loud high-pitched voice carried from one end of the long block to the other. You didn't want to be on the wrong side of her. As Mary Pat and I made our way back to the apartment after a few drinks at the bar, we stopped for a warm embrace and a very long, passionate kiss. From all the way down the block, I heard Lucille's shrill voice say, "Is this Paris?" For me at least, it was Paris and a lot more.

Settling into life in a major city can be daunting but Mary Pat adjusted to life in Manhattan much better than I expected. It probably came as a shock to her that I didn't have a cent to my name, but it didn't seem to matter. We were madly in love and enjoying the beautiful fall weather in New York. I was still playing music in Fleming's. I was glad she got to experience the place I had performed several nights a week for 12 years before it closed later that fall.

After a few weeks, it was time to pay the $700 monthly rent. I used up the money Sean had loaned me on our drive cross country. I remembered a duffle bag in my closet I used for loose change. Mary Pat looked on with curiosity as I dragged the heavy bag from the closet floor. We began counting the quarters, dimes and nickels. After twenty minutes, we had the rent money and there was plenty to put towards the following month's rent. She shook her head in disbelief and we both laughed out loud.

Mary Pat signed on with a temp agency while looking for a permanent job and within a short time was in demand with several companies, one of which was Electronic Data Systems (EDS). She was offered a full-time position as administrative assistant to one of the top executives in the company. The job helped take the financial pressure off as there was now steady money coming in. Working with a great team of people also helped her assimilate into the New York way of life. They worked hard and played hard. The company often had after-work happy hours so I also got to know her co-workers.

Not long after Mary Pat started at EDS, I became an American citizen. She couldn't come to the swearing-in since she was new in the job. I was filled with emotion as I stood in the rotunda of the imposing immigration building in lower Manhattan with countless other immigrants from every corner of the world. As I took the oath, I reflected on my journey to that point with its ups and downs. I was proud to call myself an American. I was ready to start a new chapter in my life. Later that evening, I met up with Mary Pat and her co-workers and we celebrated in style.

The Courtship

After Mary Pat's arrival in NY, our relationship progressed by leaps and bounds. We talked about getting married the following year. At some point that fall, Mary Pat went to visit family in Cincinnati with her mom. Her relatives owned a jewelry store there. She arrived back to New York with an envelope of loose diamonds. At the airport, we viewed them in awe. It made the emotions and excitement we were both feeling even more real. I picked a beautiful diamond and sent it back to Hudepohl Jewelers in Cincinnati to be formed into our engagement ring.

On December 8, less than three months after arriving in New York, I suggested that we go and watch the Christmas-tree lighting at Rockefeller Center. The streets around Rockefeller Plaza were thronged with thousands of people from all over the world. The excitement grew and just seconds before the tree was lit, I got down on one knee, produced the ring, and asked Mary Pat to marry me. She said "yes" much to my relief, and to the delight of the cheering crowds around us. The Rockefeller tree lit up in all its glory, as did my heart. That night, I was the happiest man in New York.

As we went from winter to spring, we decided to hold the wedding in Ireland. Planning a wedding from three thousand miles away was a daunting challenge but we pulled it off thanks to Mary Pat's parents and my sisters in Ireland.

During Easter, we were in Boston visiting Mary Pat's sister, Colleen. Her parents were also visiting. We all went looking at wedding dresses. After much searching, Mary Pat found the perfect gown. As she was trying the dress on, the owner of the shop said, "You must be so proud of your beautiful daughter." I was so tempted to say, "Yep, sure am. I'm going to marry her in a few months." Mary Pat didn't buy the dress since she had planned to make her own. But she did find a style and lots of ideas to incorporate into her own design. Within days she was hard at work on her beautiful wedding gown.

The Wedding

We had close to fifty guests from America join us in Ireland for the wedding. We warned them that the weather might be cold despite it being the middle of summer. But we ended up with three glorious weeks where the temperature was over 80 degrees most days. Many of our guests had to buy completely new wardrobes, but they didn't care; they were enjoying the splendor of an Ireland draped in sunshine. In the run up to our wedding day, we organized several day trips for our friends and family. We explored the wild rocky landscape of Connemara and the radiant beauty of the Aran Islands, a short boat ride from the mainland. What stands out most in my memory is the fun—or as they say in Ireland, the "craic"—on the bus. There was great story telling and as always some singing. It was a coming together of multiple generations of Mary Pat's family. Mary Pat's brother, Jim, was also on the bus. I hadn't spent much time with him previously so it was great getting to know him. He was super smart like his sisters and shared that great Shields sense of humor.

We got married August 20, 1995. Ironically, we had our reception in the Connemara Coast Hotel, formally Teach Furbo, where the Sean Fleming Band was resident fifteen years earlier. The marriage ceremony took place in beautiful Bearna Church a few miles from the reception.

Several of the people I had worked with at Fleming's were now back living in Ireland and they had their own table at the reception. It was a wonderful opportunity to reunite with those who had played such a big part in my life in New York. I also had friends whom I had grown up with in Galway. It was a great day—at least the parts of it that I can remember.

Our wedding day was spectacular in every possible way up to the point where I had too much to drink. The wedding was a once-in-a-lifetime gathering of family and friends. Halfway through the reception, my speech was slurred, and I was unsteady on my feet even during our wedding dance. I wasn't falling-down drunk, but my condition was noticeable to those who knew me well and especially to Mary Pat. It's such a shame I let the drink cloud my memory of that special day. I also know I stole some of the happiness and joy Mary Pat should have experienced on a day she had waited for all her life. I certainly wasn't the Seamus Mary Pat deserved on her wedding day.

Several of Mary Pat's co-workers and their families made their way to Ireland for the wedding, including her direct boss, John Lettko, a wonderful, energetic character and a natural-born leader. He came up to me at some point during the reception and asked if I'd be interested in doing some communications work for EDS. I think he was impressed with a speech I gave during the wedding reception—before I overindulged in the drink.

The next morning, I told Mary Pat what had happened with Lettko. She made me repeat exactly what he said. Unfortunately, the Jameson had deleted most of the conversation from my memory, so I didn't have answers to her many questions. Later that day, we figured out that Lettko did indeed talk to me about a job at EDS and he set up an interview for me upon our return to the States.

We embarked on a spectacular honeymoon the day after the wedding. We stayed at the Abbeyglen Castle Hotel in Clifden, a beautiful harbor town about fifty miles from Galway. We explored Connemara taking long walks on its beautiful beaches. One of the high points was a day trip to Inishbofin, a little piece of heaven, just off the coast near Clifden. In the evenings, we dined in the restaurant of the Abbeyglen. The nights were spent in the hotel bar. People gathered around the grand piano and sang along and danced. The first evening at the bar, Mary Pat and I were awarded a first-place medal for a dance-off. It certainly wasn't our great dancing, or at least mine, but we assumed it was because we were the honeymooners. Eventually, the bar closed and the music session moved outside to the patio where it lasted till the wee hours. The hotel manager Brian, who was a great musician, and myself entertained the party goers throughout the night.

After Connemara, we headed south to Adare Manor in County Limerick. A good friend was the manager of the spectacular hotel and he made sure we were well taken care of. We went horseback riding and explored the lush grounds of the hotel. We had what I consider to be the best meal I've ever had at the Mustard Seed Restaurant, located in a small house in the beautiful quaint village of Adare, a short walk from the hotel. We were met at the door by the host and served drinks as we looked at the menu in the small cozy sitting room. When dinner was ready, we were escorted to our table. Each course was better than the last with tastes and aromas that were totally unique. It was probably the first time in my life I experienced the pure joy of dining. I'm sure my gorgeous bride had something to do with it. Our romantic dinner was the perfect way to wind down our honeymoon. Later we sat at the bar back at the hotel and talked about our future and our dreams. I only had a few drinks and didn't have to worry about a hangover or what I said or did the night before. Sadly, that was rarely the case.

There was great excitement when we got back to Galway. Several of our American guests stayed around after the wedding to explore Ireland. We had some memorable family gatherings, once again enjoying the beautiful weather. My family got to know Mary Pat well during those three weeks. They were delighted to see me so happy and relaxed. They marveled, as many people did, at how I managed to convince such a beautiful and smart woman to marry me.

A Real Job

Two weeks later, at age 41, I walked through the doors of American Express Bank in the World Financial Center in lower Manhattan to interview for a job with EDS (the outsourcing company for the bank). Other than weddings and funerals, it was the only time I had worn a suit since my Confirmation.

After a short interview, I was offered a job as a communications consultant for EDS. This is where things get funny. Although I had a master's degree in Media Studies, I literally didn't know how to operate a copier or a fax machine. Even worse, I hadn't a clue what Microsoft Windows was, and I had taken a job as the communications guy for the second-largest information technology firm in America.

My stomach was in bits walking through the door on my first day. I felt like throwing up. I was reminded of my first day at St. Enda's and Montclair State College when I wanted to turn around and run home. Somehow, I managed to get through the day but I knew I was punching way above my belt. My biggest fear was letting Mary Pat down. In the nine months she had been with EDS, she had become an important part of their team.

Each day, I went to work with that knot in my stomach. My business writing was weak, I had zero technology skills, and I knew nothing about marketing. Thankfully, EDS hired a consultant, Bill Duncan, to help get the communications rolling on the AmEx account. Bill was an old-school sportswriter who had done consulting work for EDS for several years. I think Bill didn't believe it was possible for someone my age to be so absolutely clueless about the business world. But he saw a bit of himself in me—like Bill, I was a rebel in terms of creating my own path in life.

Some of those early days were quite dark and in some ways frightening. I was accustomed to being a relatively successful musician all my life. I played Carnegie Hall at age 24 and had been at the top of my game for over ten years at Fleming's. But I felt I could do nothing right in my day job.

I was at EDS about three months when I was asked to write a speech for one of the top executives at American Express Bank (AEB). Given my job performance to that point, I figured it was a matter of weeks before EDS were forced to let me go. Messing up a speech for a senior executive would be the last straw. I went into a conference room and told my assistant I needed to be left alone for the afternoon.

I emerged three hours later with a draft of the speech. With the blessing, and I'm sure the trepidation, of my boss, I faxed it off to the head of operations for AEB who was travelling to India to give the speech. I expected the worst but was shocked when I got a call from Mike Higgins, the EDS account executive, saying the head of operations at the bank was thrilled with the speech and only wanted one or two words changed. Higgins was a great boss and was very good to me. I surely didn't want to put him in a bad place. I was able to breathe again. In a moment, my mood changed from one of abject failure to one of hope and optimism. It was a turning point for me. Mary Pat, some of our co-workers, and I went out for drinks that evening to celebrate.

With a victory under my belt, I bought myself some time but there was work to do if I were to continue in the corporate world. My writing improved as did my tech skills. I'm a good listener, and I'm always open to criticism as long as it's constructive. Listening and learning every day from some of the immensely talented individuals on the account helped me survive those early days. I also got along great with the bank executives and that was important for the EDS leadership.

That Christmas, EDS and AEB had a joint holiday party, a very elaborate affair. The bank outsourced their IT to EDS and as part of that, approximately 200 employees transitioned to EDS. I was put in charge of entertainment since my boss knew I had been in the music business for many years. I hired Bugsy Moran and the Trouble Boys, a great band from New York. Midway through the evening, Bugsy invited me up for a song. I was nervous as to how that would be received by the audience, and in particular by the AEB and EDS leadership—most of whom didn't know I was a musician. I picked up the guitar and launched into an old blues standard. Once on stage, the nerves disappeared, and I was transported to my happy place, forgetting that these people were seeing their clueless newbie to the corporate world transform into a wild guitar player. I finished the last chord as the room erupted in applause and cheering. Before that party, I hid that I was a musician for fear I wouldn't be taken seriously. Those four minutes ripping into the guitar changed all that and the music became my ally in winning over the client.

Just When You Think Over

My run with Sean Fleming had been a good one but as our residency at his bar came to an end, I knew it was time to move on. I gave my notice to Sean not long after starting at EDS. We had travelled a long adventurous road together over a thirteen-year period. We almost broke through on the national front a few times. I had experiences with Sean that most guitar players could only dream of. We played to a packed house at Fleming's for twelve years straight and we recorded with some of the world's most talented musicians. We did festivals up and down the East Coast and the Midwest and as far away as the Czech Republic and Italy. But my musical tastes were changing and I wanted to perform with other artists. I knew nobody would approach me when I was still with Sean. He was held in high regard by all. I got a great send-off from Sean and all the fans who had followed the band through the years. I had more farewell shows than The Who.

My hiatus from music lasted all of a few months. I got a call from Blackthorn, a band based out of Philadelphia. They were having a problem with their guitarist and asked me to fill in for a night. I had seen them for the first time a few months earlier and was impressed by their full sound and their energy on stage. Despite that, I was hesitant to travel the 100 miles to Philly to do a show with a band I had never worked with. I asked Mary Pat if she was okay with me doing this once-off show and she said go for it.

I was surprised when I got to the venue to find several hundred people waiting for us to go on stage. The gig went well and I had no problem following along three hours' worth of music. The four members of the band were a lot of fun with a wonderful banter back and forth all night long. The Celtic Rock music the band played provided endless opportunities to showcase my guitar skills.

I got called again the following week to "fill in." This went on for at least six weeks and just as I was about to do my final show, the band leader Paul Moore asked me to join the band fulltime. I wasn't sure what to do. It was so much fun to be with a great band again and the crowds were getting bigger with each show. I didn't know how Mary Pat would feel about me going back to the music. She, along with her parents, were at what was to be my final show with Blackthorn down at the Jersey Shore. Mary Pat said she knew how happy I was playing with Blackthorn and she would be okay with me joining the band. Her parents were over the moon as they loved Blackthorn and the excitement building around us.

I continued to do my day job. Mary Pat and I were looking at buying a house and we were ready to start a family so the extra money from the band came in handy. Blackthorn did close to 90 shows a year. It was an exhausting schedule, but the band gave me a soft landing every Friday night after the stress of the corporate job. All the guys in the band had day jobs so we limited shows to three weekends a month.

I liked many parts of the day job, such as the people I worked with and the presence of some routine in my life. Also, I enjoyed having a regular income with health insurance for the first time in my life. I did find the politics of the corporate world hard to take. I thought the music business was cut-throat but quickly found that corporate life meant watching your back every day.

Moving on Out

After a year of living in New York, we knew it was time to move out of Manhattan. We found a lovely rental townhouse in Montclair, New Jersey, which was still an easy commute to Manhattan for work. Mary Pat was doing well at EDS and I made it past my probationary period, so life was good.

Almost exactly one year after we were married, we found out Mary Pat was pregnant. I was excited, delighted and scared to death. Before meeting Mary Pat, I was resigned to the probability I would never marry again, let alone become a dad. Now I was going to be a father for the first time at age 42 and couldn't have been happier. When Mary Pat was in the late stage of pregnancy, we bought our first house in Cranford, New Jersey. We had fallen in love with the town on first sight. With its tree-lined streets and small-town feel, I felt we were walking into a Norman Rockwell painting.

On a busy Memorial Weekend in 1997, while on stage with Blackthorn down at the New Jersey shore, I got a message on my beeper from Mary Pat saying it was time to head home as she had gone into the early stages of labor. Blackthorn did one encore and then I was in my car driving with my heart in my mouth to make sure I was at the hospital for the birth. As it turned out, we had to wait another day but was it ever worth the wait. From the moment he arrived James stole my heart. As I looked at his tiny, squirming body, it hit me Mary Pat and I were now responsible for making sure sweet baby James was given the best opportunity for a wonderful life. It never entered my head a child would bring such indescribable joy into our lives.

In the course of one week, Mary Pat gave birth to our first child, we bought a new car (yes, it was a minivan), and we moved from a rented town house in Montclair to our new home in Cranford. It was a week of utter chaos. Bringing a new baby home to a house packed up and ready to move meant James spent the first few nights of his life sleeping in a laundry basket surrounded by boxes before we had a proper nursey set up in our new home. Mary Pat's parents were a great help during that time. Her mom still worked for IBM and managed to make sure she had many business trips to the East Coast.

After several months, Mary Pat went back to work part-time at EDS. She found it hard leaving James with a babysitter, but on the other hand, she was glad to be back working with the people she had developed a great bond with.

Blackthorn's popularity continued to grow, to the point it was rare for us to play to a crowd of less than five or six hundred and often we performed to an audience of a thousand or more. To say that the band drank a lot was an understatement. During one particular gig, the bartenders had a pool to see how much we could drink in one night. They stopped counting after 75 beers. There were only five in the band at the time. The only thing that saved us was that nobody did drugs. I was the only one who drank liquor. The band was a constant for me even as my day job began to evolve.

Changes

We welcomed our second son, Rory, in November of 1998. It was an emergency cesarean section. As the doctors and nurses ran around the maternity area in a frenzy, I feared for the safety of Mary Pat and the baby. I couldn't imagine life without Mary Pat.

Shortly after the birth, Rory spent several days in hospital being monitored for an infection. Meanwhile Mary Pat was recovering from the cesarean section. It was a difficult time but once again her parents were there to help us through it.

Mary Pat left EDS to focus on raising the children not long after Rory was born. At work, many of the people I liked in my day job at EDS, including my boss Mike Higgins, had moved on. Several joined a new company called Sapient, which was doing some innovative work in the dot.com/internet world. I was recruited by a friend I had worked with at EDS and started working at Sapient as part of the marketing team in the fall of '99. It was a collegiate environment as most of the staff were under the age of forty. Employees were encouraged to explore new ideas and new ways of doing things. Everyone in the company had an opportunity to be heard. We were the rock stars of the internet and the media were paying attention to this upstart company.

Within a year and a half, I was made a director of the company and was well on the way to becoming a vice president. I was certain I would stay there until my retirement, and given the trajectory of Sapient, I would have been able to do that in ten years, if not sooner. I loved every minute of my time there. Sadly, Sapient was hit hard when the dot.com bubble burst. There were several rounds of layoffs and I was let go along with 100 others July 3, 2001. I was well taken care of financially by Sapient and decided it might be a good opportunity to take a break from corporate life.

I knew Sapient was considering mass layoffs so a week before being let go, I went back to NYU to visit my professors in the media department. I told Terry Moran, my advisor during my time at the university, I would love to teach a course at NYU. I was also interested in going back to finish the PhD I had had put on hold a few years earlier.

Dad Duty

Two hours after being let go from Sapient, I was offered an adjunct teaching position in the journalism department at NYU. A few days later, I got a call from Fordham University and they wanted me to teach a course in information technologies. The stars were aligned.

By then, our beautiful daughter Nora had arrived so we now had three children, all under the age of four. Having left the corporate world with a good steady salary, I needed to piece together multiple jobs such as teaching at NYU and Fordham and my shows with Blackthorn, but even then it was difficult to make it financially. Mary Pat took a job as a designer at an Ethan Allen store to earn much needed extra money and to get health insurance now that our COBRA (health insurance after job termination) was running out.

Mary Pat's parents had moved to Cranford around this time. On the days I wasn't teaching, I took care of the little ones. That was a massive challenge for me as I wasn't the best with young children. Mary Pat's parents helped care for the kids when we were out of pocket.

My first day taking care of all three kids by myself for a full eight-hour day was a disaster. Mary Pat gave me very specific instructions, but I was a nervous wreck, especially since Nora was only two years old. Somehow, I managed to get through the day. I was proud as could be when the children were still alive as Mary Pat walked in the door that evening. She seemed very quiet. When I asked her what was the matter, she said, "Have you looked around?" It was only then I noticed every single toy was out of the closet and toy box. Juice boxes littered the floor along with crackers and candy wrappers. The place was an absolute mess. I had a lot to learn.

September Skies

"September Skies," by Seamus Kelleher

She stood there in the garden, looking towards the sky
She had so many questions, still no reason why
When he pulled into the driveway
You could see it in his eyes
Eyewitness to hell, September Skies

I was excited to be teaching at NYU. My first class was on Tuesday, September 4, 2001. I had 250 students, mostly freshmen and sophomores. I could hear them chatting and laughing even before I entered the large oval auditorium-style classroom. I did a little part-time teaching before but had never been in front of that many students. I was used to performing to thousands of people with Blackthorn, so I wasn't too intimated. That first session was exhilarating, and I couldn't wait for class the following week. The course was called "Television and the Information Explosion." I used the history of television news as the narrative for the class. I had no idea how poignant the class would become within just a few days.

On the morning of September 11, 2001, I was scheduled to go to NYU regarding some paperwork for my re-enrollment in the PhD program. I held off going into the city until noon to avoid the heavy traffic. I was scrolling through the news on my computer in the morning when I saw something about a plane hitting the North Tower of the World Trade Center. Initially, I thought it was just a small plane accidently glancing off the side of the tower. I knew from working there that several small aircraft passed close by the hundred-plus-story towers each day.

It didn't take long to see that something was terribly wrong when at 9:03 am, live on TV, a second plane crashed into the South Tower of the World Trade Center. I immediately called Mary Pat in so she could see what was happening. It was apparent after a few minutes we were witnessing a catastrophe unfold in front of our eyes. It was made all the more chilling because I had worked in the World Financial Center adjacent to the Towers and Mary Pat had worked in 7 World Trade.

We knew every inch of the area. When we worked at EDS, I organized events at Windows of the World atop the World Trade Center, and Mary Pat and I often met for lunch in the maze of restaurants in the tunnels beneath the Towers.

We had that sinking feeling inside of not knowing if this was just the beginning of a larger attack on New York City and indeed other cities across America. My gut reaction was to prepare for the worst. As soon as the first Tower collapsed, I said to Mary Pat, "We need some supplies." In the local supermarket, I found many like myself grabbing water and other basics. On my way home, I heard a stunned newscaster on the car radio, his voice wavering in disbelief, say the second tower collapsed. The scenes being described were horrifying—people leaping to their deaths sometimes holding hands from both Towers—people waving in utter despair from the roofs of the Towers before they collapsed. We wondered how many people we knew were being impacted directly by this horrific carnage.

It's ironic that the tragedy occurred on what was probably the most beautiful day of the year. The sun was shining brightly in a cloudless blue sky in Cranford and a gentle cool breeze kept the temperature at an even 70 degrees. The beauty of the day and the horror that unfolded just twenty miles away from our home made for a chilling juxtaposition.

After several hours of watching the tragedy unfold on TV, I had to get away from it for a while. My anxiety level was rising by the minute. I decided to put a tar sealant on our driveway in a futile attempt to keep my mind off what was happening. A short while later, Mary Pat and I were talking with our neighbor, Kelly, from the house directly across the street, when her husband, Dave, pulled into their driveway. He worked in the Bank of America building, directly across from the fallen Towers. He made it out safely and was one of the lucky ones who quickly got out of Manhattan before all the arteries out of the city became clogged with those trying to escape the mayhem.

Dave was covered in a grey dust from the falling debris. He had a look of fear in his eyes I'll never forget. He always came across as a tough guy, brimming with confidence. He was part of the local EMS volunteer squad and had seen a lot of emergency situations. But this was different. He held his wife tightly. Without a word, Mary Pat grabbed their two little girls and took them down the street to a neighbor's house for a birthday party so Kelly and Dave could have time to themselves. That scenario was played out that day in small towns like ours all over New Jersey, New York and Connecticut. Sadly, many didn't make it home, including six people from Cranford. Our town was small, so everyone knew someone who had suffered a loss.

I'm glad our children were too young to understand what was happening. Our two oldest, James and Rory, were playing with their Rescue Hero toys when James said, "Dad, Billy Blazes will help." The Rescue Hero Billy Blazes helped people escape fires and other disasters, and I think that's when it all hit me. We lost too many Billy Blazes on 9/11, not just in New York but at the Pentagon in Washington, DC, and in Shanksville, Pennsylvania.

The next several days were very difficult. We tried to keep life as normal as possible for the sake of the children. At every turn, there were stories of bravery, tragedy, sacrifice and loss. We put a limit on the amount of time we watched the news on TV. We were paralyzed by the heart-wrenching images and the unimaginable suffering. It was too much.

I was supposed to have class at NYU on the 12th of September, but the university closed for over a week and I didn't go into New York until the following week. Nothing prepared me for what I witnessed. As I approached the Holland Tunnel, I teared up as I saw the huge gaping hole in the skyline I had known and loved since coming to America in 1974.

I parked my car a few blocks from NYU. The acrid smoke from the still-smoldering fire lingered in the air. It was uncomfortable to breathe. An eerie quiet had descended over the entire city. The hustle and bustle and the sound of laughter on the streets of the city, characteristic of a typical September day, were replaced by sadness and emptiness. People's faces on the subway were ashen. They wondered what was next—was this just the beginning—was it Armageddon?

On September 18, I walked back into my classroom at NYU. Gone was the joyous laughter, the flirting, the smiles. All I could hear was occasional sobbing that emanated from all sides of the room. Looking out from my lectern, I saw over two hundred terrified individuals who had their innocence ripped from them in just a few short minutes.

I was determined to keep things as normal as possible for the students. I figured I could talk about the media coverage of the tragedy since that aligned to the content of my syllabus. I asked how many had watched events unfold on TV and was surprised to see only a few nod their heads. A few more hands went up when I asked who had seen it on the internet. It was only then I realized most of the students watched the whole thing unfold in person. Many of them were living in an NYU dorm a few blocks from the Towers. The rest of them were less than a mile away on campus and saw the buildings collapse from their dorm windows.

What do you say to a group of people in their late teens who witnessed first-hand the horror of such a tragedy? One day they were celebrating a life full of promise and opportunity, now their world was shattered. I said time would allow the scars of 9/11 to heal and promised them that despite their heavy hearts and the tears, there would be laughter in our classroom before the end of the semester.

I told them when I was just ten years old growing up in Ireland, the assassination of John F. Kennedy made us all wonder what lay ahead. Kennedy was the man who saved the world from total destruction during the Cuban missile crisis. He was going to end the Vietnam War and finally deal with the racial injustice that was tearing America apart. Kennedy had just visited Ireland a few months before his death. I told them of that horrible feeling of hopelessness we felt as a nation. It took time, but eventually we moved forward.

For several weeks after 9/11, I was more of a counselor than a teacher. Gradually, over the course of the semester, the students did indeed begin to smile again and laugh at my silly jokes. During my classes at Fordham University, I had a similar experience. But our world had changed, we were all different after that terrible September day.

A few weeks after the tragedy, I brought Mary Pat into the city. She heard me talk about what I saw in Manhattan, but it was something she needed to experience for herself. For that first few weeks after 9/11, she was focused on making sure the children were okay; now it was her turn to mourn.

We went to the site of the fallen Towers, or Ground Zero as it was now known. We were deeply moved by what we witnessed—the mangled remains of the Towers with white smoke still billowing from the twisted wreckage. We didn't say a word as we looked at the makeshift memorials scattered all over the side streets of lower Manhattan. We passed a firehouse and realized from handmade signs left outside on the sidewalk that several firefighters from that squad lost their lives running into the Towers before they collapsed. All I could say was "thank you" to a lone member of the squad standing in the doorway. My words seemed so inadequate, so shallow, but I wanted to show my appreciation for his bravery and the heroism of his fellow firefighters who were lost on that awful day.

There were thousands of flyers with photos of missing people posted all over lower Manhattan. Families were hanging on to hope a loved one miraculously made it out of the devastation alive and might be in one of the surrounding hospitals in the tri-state area. It was gut wrenching and I could tell Mary Pat's heart was breaking as we walked through the silent streets.

The weeks rolled by, and we all dealt with the grief in our own way. As the shock of 9/11 wore off, I began feeling very depressed for the first time in years. The depression was accompanied by anxiety about the future. What would happen if I was at NYU and there was another attack—was this the beginning of a new kind of war—would things ever return to normal—what did the future hold for my children in this changed world?

Blackthorn was finishing up a new album in the weeks immediately following 9/11 and that helped me navigate through those dark days. We recorded the album in Woodstock, New York, during the summer but we were mixing and dubbing some instruments in Philly. It served as a distraction for us all.

Three weeks after 9/11, Blackthorn headlined a big festival in Wildwood at the Jersey Shore. Known as Irish Weekend, it was an annual event where close to a quarter million people converged on the small Jersey Shore town to celebrate their Irish heritage. Blackthorn was the main attraction during the three-day festival performing at Moore's Inlet overlooking the wild Atlantic. The normal capacity at Moore's was 500 but for the festival weekend, they erected an elaborate marquee that could accommodate 5,000 people. Over the course of 72 hours, we did 10 hour-long shows, always performing to a full tent.

We seriously questioned the wisdom of doing the festival so soon after 9/11, but we all agreed people needed to come together during such a difficult time. When we walked on stage for our first show, we could see the emotion on people's faces. It was as if they were holding in a terrible sadness and pain. For many, seeing their beloved Blackthorn gave them hope. We represented something normal in abnormal times. I was never prouder of our band than I was that weekend. Over the three days, we played to over 50,000 people and mourned the loss of our fellow citizens. We also celebrated life and our Irish culture and provided hope for our audience and ourselves we would indeed emerge from the fog of 9/11.

As the months rolled on, I found it hard to concentrate on my course work for the PhD. Midway through the spring semester, I decided I couldn't pursue the doctorate any further. My heart wasn't in it anymore. I needed to step back. It was a difficult decision as I was three-quarters of the way through the program. But I knew it was the right thing to do and immediately felt some relief.

I was trying to be strong for Mary Pat, the kids and my students at NYU and Fordham, but I was suffering inside. I found it hard to get out of bed in the mornings and was full of fear when driving to work or getting on the New York subway. I was sad all the time. Knowing what I know now, I believe I was suffering some form of Post-Traumatic Stress Disorder (PTSD). With the benefit of hindsight, I should have gotten professional help. During my life, I've been pretty good at recognizing the signs when my mental health was in decline—sadness, lack of hope, sleeping all day, lack of joy, inability to engage with family and friends. But not this time. For several months I was in an incredibly dark place often using alcohol to blur the pain.

Thanks to an increased focus on my music, the teaching at NYU and Fordham that I enjoyed so much and the support of Mary Pat, after several months I was able to dig myself out of the darkness. I also had three beautiful children who brought me joy even on the saddest of days.

Songs & Stories

As time passed, my mood was up and down. While I was busy with the teaching, the childcare, and my shows with Blackthorn, I needed a lift. One morning out of nowhere, a crazy idea popped into my head. It was a rare moment of clarity during an otherwise difficult time. For years I had been talking to Mary Pat about doing a show to celebrate the life of my guitar hero Rory Gallagher, who passed away in 1995 at age 47. Rory was a world-renowned blues guitar player and a terrific songwriter. He was one of Bob Dylan's favorite guitar players. Jimi Hendrix, Muddy Waters, John Lennon and Brian May also loved his playing and counted him as one of the world's top players. I met him when I was a teenager and had the good fortune to see him perform many times. I asked him about his influences and how he practiced. He inspired me to be the best guitarist I could be. He was truly a beautiful human being.

When I mentioned my idea of doing a show this time, Mary Pat said, "Don't just talk about it; pick a date and do it." With her full support, I had a renewed focus and set about putting together the show. I flew to Reading in the UK to visit my friend Brendan Glynn who was fighting a battle with pancreatic cancer. Pierce Turner, an extraordinary singer/songwriter and a good friend, put me in touch with Rory's brother, Donal, who lived in London and handled Rory's estate. Brendan and I met with Donal and I asked him for permission to do a show in New York to celebrate Rory's life and music. I made a mock-up poster and presented him with the script I intended to use during the show. I called the show Songs & Stories: New York Remembers Rory Gallagher. Donal was impressed by my presentation and the work I put into it. He was incredibly gracious and gave me the rights to do the show. He said he couldn't promise, but he would try and make it to New York for the concert.

Brendan enjoyed our visit with Donal as he was also a huge Rory Gallagher fan. On the way back to Reading on the train, Brendan and I reminisced, talking about every girl we had ever met growing up in Galway. His wife Sue told me after Brendan passed that he enjoyed our two days together like it was a faraway vacation. I loved him like a brother. That was the last time I saw him.

With the help of my good buddy, Larry Kirwan (the lead singer with the hugely successful Celtic Rock band Black 47), I was able to secure the Bottom Line Club, a world famous venue located on West 4th Street in the middle of the NYU campus. Rory played there many times as had the likes of Bruce Springsteen, Eric Clapton and Dolly Parton.

I enlisted the help of another guitar player and good friend, Justin Jordan, to help produce the show. Justin is a great player and also a huge Rory fan. I also called on my long-time friend Chris Ebneth to play bass and Brian (Bugsy) Moran to do keyboards. The final link in the chain was Jonathan Mover, one of the world's finest drummers.

The idea behind Songs & Stories was to ask several singers I worked and recorded with over the years to do their own interpretation of a few Rory songs. I called on Pierce Turner, Larry Kirwan, Pat McGuire, Brian Moran (Bugsy) and Sean Fleming to make the magic happen. A week into the production, I woke up panicked, realizing I had stepped way out of my comfort zone. All I could think of was all that might go wrong. Could I really pull this off?

In spring of 2002, Mary Pat was hoping to add one more to our family. We were still struggling financially but I agreed that we'd give it a few

241

months but if we weren't pregnant by summer we would stop trying and count our blessings. The summer ended without Mary Pat being pregnant. Part of me was relieved but I knew Mary Pat wanted another child. After returning from a long rehearsal two weeks before the show at the Bottom Line, Mary Pat wasn't herself. I asked if her mood had anything to do with still wanting another child. She started sobbing. I said, "Are you pregnant?" The crying got worse. I just started laughing and said, "Let's celebrate." She looked at me in disbelief and said, "I know you're not ready for another child." I stopped her mid-sentence and said, "That was five minutes ago. This is a new reality now so let's just embrace it and celebrate." I pulled a small bottle of champagne from the fridge and poured two glasses to toast the good news. I had a few glasses and Mary Pat had one sip.

I needed money desperately to stage and promote "Songs & Stories." I turned to Danny McDonald, the bartender from the Green Derby, and Mike Jewel, whom I worked with in Fleming's for years. They had opened two successful bars in lower Manhattan. I met with them and explained in detail what I wanted to do at the Bottom Line. I could see that familiar smile on their faces. They knew me well and saw the passion and love I had for Rory—something they both shared. Without hesitation, they said, "How much?" The financial support from Mike and Danny took a weight off my shoulders and allowed me to focus on the execution of the show. I was humbled by the respect they had for me.

The script I wrote for the show included many stories about Rory, his music and his life. I felt such a responsibility to do justice to Rory and his work. This was the first American tribute to Rory and his brother was scheduled to fly in from London.

A Zen-like calm descended on me the day of the show. It happens a lot when I have a major occurrence in my life. Maybe it's just my defense mechanisms kicking in so I can execute my often over-the-top daft ideas.

I didn't know what to expect crowd-wise on the night of the concert. The Bottom Line held over four hundred people, but I would have been happy with two hundred. The show sold out. Just before curtain time, the owner of the Bottom Line, Allan Pepper, brought Donal Gallagher backstage to see me. He had a huge smile on his face. As I went to shake hands, Donal put his arms around me and gave me a long hug. Even before the first note sounded, he knew how much work I put into the inaugural tribute to the brother he loved so much.

The lights came on at 8 pm to a roar from the crowd. As I walked on stage, the significance of the night dawned on me. I was doing a show to honor one of the greatest guitar players the world had ever seen and his brother was there to support me. I started the show with an audio recording of a show Rory did at the Bottom Line in 1976. For the next two hours, I was taken to somewhere I had never been before. I told stories about Rory and introduced each artist. Everything worked like clockwork. My nerves dissipated after a few minutes. My confidence took a giant leap with the great reaction from the audience to each artist and their songs.

Halfway through the show, I invited Donal on stage to say a few words about his brother. He thanked me for putting on the show and said Rory would have been privileged to play with the musicians on stage at the Bottom Line that night. I was humbled when he presented me with the official Irish Rory Gallagher stamp that was issued in Ireland that very day. In a way, Song & Stories was an opportunity for me to say thanks for the kindness Rory had shown a young seventeen-year-old guitar player and the inspiration he provided me back in the early '70s.

243

Each artist performed to perfection during the two-hour show. It was awe inspiring to hear what they did with the songs I assigned to them. We did one encore as that was all we had left and got a standing ovation that seemed to go on forever.

I went out into the audience to say goodbye to a pregnant Mary Pat and her folks who were about to head home. Mary Pat knew how hard I worked to make this happen and she was delighted for me.

I was being congratulated by people I had never met before. It was only then I realized people had come from as far away as Holland and California to be part of the evening. Nobody wanted to leave the Bottom Line. Many of them knew each other from attending the same Rory shows over the years. They had been waiting a long time to come together and celebrate their beloved Rory Gallagher.

I was deeply engaged in conversation with an ardent Rory fan when one of the bouncers said, "Pepper wants to see you." I said, "Just a minute" but he said "Now" as if I was being commanded by royalty. Given the tone of voice, I expected some bad news. I went into Pepper's tiny, cluttered office. He had developed a reputation in New York as tough to deal with but we got along well. I wondered how many great artists and their agents had stepped into that office over the years. Pepper said, "Seamus, this was one of the best shows at the Bottom Line in recent years." I was shocked and felt instant relief. He said I created something very special and was welcome to come back at any time in the future regardless of what type of show I wanted to produce. He complimented me on my professionalism before and during the concert, and said the staff were amazed I had handed them a script during rehearsal. He said that didn't happen too often at the Bottom Line.

After many more conversations with the Rory faithful, I walked the streets of lower Manhattan with Donal Gallagher the few blocks to the post-concert reception hosted by Danny McDonald and Mike Jewel. It was supposed to be just for the artists and their families, but Danny and Mike, in their usual spirit of generosity, opened it up to everyone. It was a wonderful gesture and afforded those who had travelled so far an opportunity to mingle and share more Rory stories. Everyone was buzzing about the evening. Monty Monaghan, a great mandolin player who was part of the show, said, "This is one of the best nights of my life, Seamus." I smiled and said, "For me too, Monty."

As Mary Pat was leaving the Bottom Line, she said, "Don't overdo it; this is a special night for you." I knew she was hoping I wouldn't let alcohol ruin a great evening. For once, I took her advice and only had two drinks and was able to enjoy and savor every moment.

The owner of Fitzpatrick's Hotel in midtown Manhattan was generous enough to provide Donal and myself with complimentary hotel rooms. We made our way back there after the post-concert reception. Here I was walking the streets of New York at 5 am with the brother of my guitar hero Rory Gallagher and he was saying this was one of the best-ever tributes to his brother. I was in seventh heaven.

After a few hours of sleep, Donal and I met for breakfast in the hotel lobby before he left for a TV interview and I to run a few blocks to the Fordham University Manhattan Campus where I had to teach a class. I needed something to bring me back to reality. I told the students what had unfolded the night before and to forgive me if I seemed a bit loopy.

When I finally got home to New Jersey that night, I logged on to my email and was overwhelmed by the positive feedback from my friends and supporters. The show had touched many people. Some thanked me for allowing them to celebrate the life and music of Rory who they held so dear. Others said they saw another side of me during the show, where I was center stage rather than being confined to the background as was the case with Sean Fleming and Blackthorn. Songs & Stories got some great reviews in the New York Irish papers with Mike Farragher, a well-known music critic from the *Irish Voice,* calling it one of the best Irish shows of the decade.

The magic that happened at the Bottom Line was captured on film by Victor Zimet and Stephanie Silber, a husband-and-wife movie-making team. Larry Kirwan put me in touch with them. Even after telling Vic and Steph I had no money to pay them, they decided it was important to document the evening on film. Not only that, but they filmed some of the rehearsals and captured the artists' excitement about the project. The end result of Vic and Steph's efforts was a beautiful documentary: Songs & Stories: New York Remembers Rory Gallagher. It was shown at some film festivals and broadcast on Irish Television. Most important of all, it's something that everyone involved in the show has to remind them of that special evening at the Bottom Line in October 2002.

I was forty-eight when I did the show at the Bottom Line. That one night changed my life. Before then, I was afraid to take on big projects for fear of depression and anxiety getting in the way. By executing Songs & Stories with all its complexities and moving parts, I knew I could do more with my God-given talent. I was no longer the sideman for Sean Fleming or Blackthorn. I was ready to forge my own destiny.

A Gift

Things continued to be tight on the financial front for Mary Pat and me. There was still no steady day job. I was working hard teaching at Fordham and NYU and performing each weekend with Blackthorn, but the lack of health benefits and a consistent paycheck took its toll. By this time, Mary Pat had left Ethan Allen due to the difficult hours that the retail work demanded and immediately started her own drapery business Kelleher Creations. It was a bold move, especially with three children under the age of five and another one on the way. But Mary Pat is a tireless worker. I knew her business would blossom, but it would take a while.

Aidan came into our lives in May 2003. Maybe I'm romanticizing it now, but it seems like he had a smile on his face from day one. Since Mary Pat's business was picking up and there was no such thing as maternity leave for your own small business, I was actively involved in taking care of Aidan from day one—more so than any of the other children. He was the gift I wasn't expecting and the gift kept on giving.

A few weeks after his birth, Mary Pat had an appointment with a new client, so I was in charge of the kids. As she prepared for work, I held Aidan on my shoulder, making a cup of Maxwell House instant coffee using just one hand, and helping get James, Rory and Nora get ready for the day. Mary Pat looked at me and said, "Boy, you've come a long way." It was only a few years earlier that I was afraid of being left alone for a minute with any of the kids. When Mary Pat came home from work, unlike the first time I was alone with the children, the house was in relatively good working order with the toys put back where they belonged, and the Cheerios and juice boxes cleared from the kitchen floor.

I was sure my guitar playing would suffer with the arrival of Aidan. Babies need a lot of minding. I know it's crazy to think of something like that as you await the birth of a child, but the mind of a musician is not the most rational in the world. But I ended up having more time than ever to focus on my guitar playing. Aidan went down for a two-hour nap like clockwork every morning at 9 am while James was in kindergarten and Rory in preschool. Nora was home but she entertained herself, so I had plenty of practice time. After several months, I could see my playing improving dramatically. That year, I attended several workshops with some of the world's best pickers, including Tommy Emmanuel, Pete Huttlinger and Richard Smith. In many ways, the birth of Aidan was a factor in me being reborn as a guitar player.

Risking it All

Despite all the good that was happening in my life with the birth of Aidan and my revitalized passion for guitar, I was drinking a lot. I often went for days without even thinking about a drink, but then I'd attend an event and get totally intoxicated. It was a strange kind of drinking and it scared Mary Pat. More than once, I got into my car, sometimes with loved ones, when I shouldn't have. Of all the things I have done in my life, that is what I regret most. I never got pulled over for drunk driving and, to the best of my knowledge, I never hit anyone, but that doesn't absolve me from my actions.

The drinking had a devastating impact on my relationship with Mary Pat. The only times I ever remember her raising her voice during our 25 years of marriage were when I walked in the door after driving the car when drunk. I had nothing to say when she got angry with me and that made things even worse. I knew I was in the wrong and just had a blank stare on my face. An uncomfortable silence followed those episodes that often lasted for days. I was full of remorse and shame and vowed it would never happen again. Sadly, it did. I was risking it all.

Mary Pat was working hard to make her sewing business a success while taking care of four young children. She didn't have a minute to herself. I put her through hell, and I was doing nothing to change that. I came home one afternoon after having drinks over lunch in Manhattan with some friends. As I was leaving the parking garage in the city, I damaged the door of the minivan. When Mary Pat saw the shape I was in and the damage to the minivan, she almost put her fist through the wall. Rightly so, she yelled at me. There was a look of terror on her face I'd never seen before. She asked me how I could be so stupid and inconsiderate to endanger other people's lives and my own by getting on the road drunk. I didn't have an answer.

After each drunken occurrence, I tried to moderate my drinking, often not touching it for weeks on end. Then I'd have one drink when out with Mary Pat to show her I was in control. But I never was, and after a few weeks, one drink became two or three and there was no off switch.

Back to Work

I got some part-time work with a marketing company in New Jersey called Kinesis. It was three days a week but it was good to be working with a company again. I also started writing a weekly column for a New York-based Irish paper the *Irish Examiner*. The publisher, Paddy McCarthy, gave me free rein to write about whatever I wanted. It was challenging meeting a weekly deadline, but my writing improved dramatically as a result. It also got me reconnected with the Irish community. In addition, one of my neighbors in Cranford, Larry Kain, asked me to write articles for his magazine *The Hometown Quarterly*.

So now I was working a few days a week, teaching at NYU, writing for a newspaper and a magazine, and also playing with the band in Philadelphia. My biggest challenge was keeping track of where I needed to be on a given day. Mary Pat's business was taking off. She moved from a relatively small workroom in her mother's home to a commercial space and hired two additional employees. The new workroom wasn't far from the house and had plenty of space that allowed Mary Pat to work unconventional hours to accommodate the needs of the children. Mary Pat, being as imaginative as she is, found ways to create all kinds of adventures for the kids in the workroom using fabric remnants and the boxes that her drapery supplies came in. Aidan spent hours roller skating around the worktables while she worked when the other children were in school.

The marketing role at Kinesis led to a full-time job with one of their clients, Management Recruiters International (MRI), a franchise organization with over 600 offices worldwide. I worked in their corporate headquarters, located in Philadelphia. We provided training, business guidance and marketing to the franchisees.

Two weeks after I started at MRI, the president was fired. I was shocked and frustrated as I thought I had finally landed on my feet. The new president, Michael Jalbert, replaced most of the marketing staff and I was sure I was on the hit list. I walked into his office and said, "Michael, we both know I'm a dead man walking but you are contracted to pay me for two months. Why don't I do what I can for you and if you're not happy, we'll call it quits." He was stunned as most people feared him, but I was honest, and he seemed to like that. Co-workers were dropping like flies, but I kept doing the best work I could. During our conversation I mentioned I was an adjunct professor at NYU. He said he was taking his daughter on a college tour of the university that weekend.

That Friday when Jalbert was leaving the office, I handed him a folder with a few pages of useful background information on NYU I knew he wouldn't get on the tour of the school. He was very appreciative, and after that, he stopped by my office most days to say hello and we chatted about everything from family to the state of the economy. He was intrigued that I was teaching at NYU, playing in a band and still holding down a full-time job.

Over the course of the next few months, Jalbert and I developed a most unlikely friendship. I started writing all his communications, as well as his first major speech to the company. He liked what I was doing. I was nearing the conclusion of my contract with MRI when he asked if I would like to continue with the organization. I was made full time with the company December 2006.

It was during that period that I decided that if I didn't do a solo CD then, I probably never would. Mary Pat encouraged me to go for it. Pete Huttlinger, a world-class guitar player from whom I had taken workshops and guitar lessons, agreed to produce my record but I had to do it in Nashville where he lived. The price tag for the album was $18,000, a large sum of money I didn't have. I sent an email to family and friends offering shares in the record at $2,500 a piece. Within three days I raised over $10,000 dollars. I got a few small donations and then one day my neighbor from down the street, Scott Taylor, arrived up to the house with a check. I thought it was for $250 but nearly fell over when I realized it was for $2,500. I was equally bowled over when I got an email from two good friends in Ireland— Damien Hanley, my first guitar teacher, and Marco Magliocco, a teenage friend and supporter of my music—who got together and decided to split a share. I was taken by the support of so many. By mid-March I had raised most of the money.

I booked the studio in Nashville for the week after Easter 2007. I was determined to do mostly original songs but I was fearful of embarrassing myself in front of some of Nashville's elite musicians. It was a big risk and there was a lot of money at stake. I also felt an obligation to those who invested in the album. I reminded myself of what I had accomplished at the Bottom Line just a few years earlier. It was the right time.

With a few weeks to go before the recording in Nashville, I was short by $7,500. I figured I might need a loan. I called my friends Danny McDonald and Mike Jewel, who had helped me with my Rory show at the Bottom Line a few years previously. I didn't even get to explain the entire project. Once again they said, "How much?" and within two hours they handed me a large sum of cash with no strings attached. I was speechless.

The day before I left for Nashville, I was writing a speech for Jalbert at MRI. He was curious about my trip to Nashville and the recording process. He asked how I was fixed financially. I told him there was one share left unsold, but I could come up with the money by getting a loan. Without saying a word, he wrote a check for $2,500 and handed it to me. All I could say in my stupor was, "I suppose you won't be firing me any time soon." He put his hands on my shoulder and said, "Go get them, Seamus, and be yourself."

Four Cups of Coffee

"Four Cups of Coffee." by Seamus Kelleher

Four cups of coffee, three shots of gin,
two Irish Coffees, can't you see the shape I'm in.
Hey bartender, don't give me any more,
can't you see the devil, he's knocking at the door.

I packed my guitars and amps in my car the next day. It was a lovely crisp Saturday spring morning with the sun shining brightly. I kissed Mary Pat and hugged the kids before heading south on the fourteen-hour drive to Nashville. I made a rough demo of the songs to listen to on the way. Driving through beautiful West Virginia with its lush hills and mountains and the trees beginning to bloom, I listened to my songs and wondered what they would sound like on my way home a week later.

I arrived in Nashville late Saturday night and booked into a hotel near the studio. I was nervous at the thought of the recording process. The next day, I met with the producer Pete Huttlinger to go over the songs and discuss how we would approach them. He was a gentle soul with that wonderful gift of bringing out the very best in people.

Much to Pete's horror, I invited Andrew Harkins, a bass player from New York, to join me for the recording. Andrew is one of the most talented musicians I have ever known, but Pete was mad as hell. He had already hired the best session players in Nashville. To put Pete's mind at ease I said, "If you don't like Andrew's playing, you can bring in whoever you want. I'll pay them and I will still pay Andrew as a consultant to me."

After the rather tense exchange with Pete, I headed out to downtown Nashville to hear some music and clear my head. There was no cover charge in the honky tonk bars along Broadway, so I went from one joint to another, with my jaw open wide at the standard of music I was hearing. I kept asking myself, "What the hell are you doing here Seamus?"

Andrew showed up later that evening and we had dinner. I was so glad to have someone to share my Nashville experience with although I was praying he and Pete would get along. I didn't share Pete's concerns.

I got to Quad Studios at 9:30 am on Monday morning as requested by Pete. The studio, formerly Quadraphonic Studios, was where Neil Young recorded his iconic Harvest album. It was on Music Row, a series of closely-knit streets with dozens of world-class recording studios. In essence, Music Row is the Wall Street of the music world. Musicians were getting out of cars and vans going into what looked like normal neighborhood houses with guitars, banjos, drums and every other instrument you could imagine. For me, this was Disneyland. It was where dreams came true and where others were dashed. I was about to step on the wildest ride of my life.

Within twenty minutes of entering the studio, we were recording the first track for the album. I could tell Pete was still pissed about my bass player Andrew being there, but always the gentleman, he pretended everything was okay. We started with a simple song I had written called "Missing My Hometown."

The drummer John Gardner was simply amazing. His tempo was like a clock ticking in perfect time, but his playing was full of emotion. He was a gentle southern boy. You wouldn't know it to talk to him that he had toured with just about everyone including the Dixie Chicks.

Jeff Taylor, the keyboard player, defied belief in terms of his musicianship. Every time I turned around he was playing a different instrument. He was hired primarily as a piano player but played beautiful haunting flute and accordion the likes of which you might hear at a session somewhere in a pub in the west of Ireland. By noon, with three tracks complete, the band adjourned for lunch. We were joined by the studio manager who was also Garth Brooks' bass player. It was fun hearing all his great Nashville stories. I had to pinch myself as a reminder of what was happening.

It was back to the studio after lunch for a hectic four hours of recording. At one point, we were in the control room listening to a playback of a track when the drummer walked in saying in his droll southern accent, "It ain't right what that New York boy there is able to do on that bass guitar." Everyone agreed that Andrew was an amazing player. Pete Huttlinger finally joined in singing Andrew's praises. I'm sure he was still mad at me for my arrogance in bringing a bass player from New York to Nashville, but he quickly recognized Andrew's talent and his absolute professionalism. I felt enormous relief.

After the first day's recording, Andrew turned in early, but I was wired to the moon. I headed out to a well-known Nashville club One Station Plaza where my keyboard player, Jeff Taylor, was playing with the Time Jumpers, a country swing-type band. The Station Inn was an intimate venue that reminded me of a smaller version of the Bottom Line in New York. The band was amazing. At one point, the leader said, "Y'all, I'd like to bring a friend of the band to the stage, now please put your hands together for Vince Gill." Up gets this guy sitting behind me in blue jeans, a checkered plaid shirt, and a baseball cap.

I was absolutely floored by Gill's voice and realized this was another Nashville moment to add to my collection. He walked by me on the way back to his seat, put his hand on my shoulder and said, "How're ya doin', buddy." I nearly fell off the chair. I ran out to the car and grabbed my camera. At the end of the evening, I got my photo taken with Vince. As I left the Station Inn, it was clear I made the right decision in making my first solo album in such a magical place where just about everyone was involved in the music business. My dreams were already coming true.

On Tuesday, I was ready to rock knowing we had already several tracks under our belt. I told Pete I met Vince and he showed only mild interest. Turns out his wife, Erin, was Vince's publicist. Pete had been to Vince's house many times. The wind went out of my sails pretty quickly. I couldn't even impress Pete after meeting one of the great legends of country music. Name dropping doesn't get you too far in Nashville.

Everything went great on the Tuesday until we started recording a Rory Gallagher song "What's Going On." I couldn't get the song to work in terms of rhythm and for the first time during the recording process, I got really down. I was embarrassed in front of these super talented musicians. I asked everyone to leave the room for a while so I could try and figure it out. The drummer said, "Seamus, let's try this a different way." After a few minutes, we fixed the problem. The next take is what's on the album and it turned out to be one of the best tracks. I regained my confidence, thanks in large part to the encouragement from the drummer and him seeing I had the talent to pull this off with a little coaxing.

That night Andrew and I went out for a few pints of Guinness at an Irish bar near the studio. We knew the CD was turning into something special and we celebrated the work we did together. Andrew is a beautiful human being and he knew exactly the excitement I was feeling seeing my music come to life. Neither of us are big talkers so we sat there, enjoying the ambiance and savoring the moment.

The third day at Quad Studios was mainly reserved for my electric guitar playing. I set up my guitar and amp and let rip with "Dust My Broom," an old blues song by Robert Johnson popularized by Elmore James. The engineer and the musicians on the session were in shock seeing the quiet Seamus morph into a rocker. I could see them through the thick studio glass shaking their heads, pointing their fingers as if to say, "Look at this guy," and laughing. I certainly got their attention. When I get an electric guitar in my hands, a metamorphosis takes place. It's one of the few areas of music where I know I can go head-to-head with anyone. I think I had earned the respect of the musicians and studio staff before I started on the electric, but I grew in stature after the first take of "Dust My Broom." When I saw that wonderful approving grin on Pete Huttlinger's face, I knew I had moved the needle.

The final day of recording was reserved for mixing the songs so I'd have something to listen to on my way back home. At three in the afternoon, I walked out of Quad Studio with a rough mix of my CD. I promised myself I wouldn't listen to it until I was driving back to New Jersey the following day. But patience is a virtue I struggle with. I put the demo in the CD player of my rented car as soon as I left the studio parking lot. I got emotional when I heard the first few chords of the album's opening track, "My Friend Ben." The song is about my lifelong friend Brendan Glynn who passed from cancer a few years earlier. I felt the song did justice to our beautiful 35-year friendship. As I listened to each song, I knew I had stretched my talent to its very limit. I wanted everyone I knew to hear what I had done.

Brush with Royalty

No sooner had I gotten to my hotel when I got a call from Pete saying, "Seamus, would you like to go to a birthday party?" I was exhausted but still buzzing from listening to the rough mixes, so I said, "Sure, but who's it for?" "It's Vince Gill's fiftieth today, so that's where we're headed."

I called my sister Toni in Ireland which was cruel as I knew she was a huge country fan. "Fuck," was all I heard on the other side of the phone. The reaction from Mary Pat was similar except without the profanity. Mary Pat would have been a lot more familiar with Vince Gill than me.

Pete and I drove over to Vince's house in the early evening. His wife Erin was there all afternoon helping prepare for the event. We were met at the door by Vince's beautiful wife, Amy Grant. She welcomed Pete with open arms as she knew him well. Pete introduced me and she gave me a great big hug and said, "Seamus, congratulations on your new album; you'll have to play for us later?" Amy was even more beautiful in person than on her album covers. I have no recollection of what I said to her as I was totally star struck.

I dropped my jacket in their living room and headed out to the backyard with Pete and Amy. We were met by my new best friend, Vince. I wished him a happy birthday and he said, "Hey buddy, we had our photo taken together at the Station Inn on Monday." Nashville's biggest star remembered me. I had arrived.

In the middle of the yard, there was a bar set up and a taco stall along with a dessert bar. That was it—nothing over the top. The focus for the evening was on a tent with chairs set up all around a small stage. For the next three hours, I witnessed some of the best music I've ever heard. Janis

Ian got up and sang as did Don Schlitz, the guy who wrote "The Gambler." He sang it not as the popularized version from Kenny Rogers but as a beautiful ballad.

It struck me that the party was all about these singer/songwriters. There were very few if any of the typical Nashville celebrities in the crowd. Vince wanted to celebrate with the people who write the music. Amy also got up and sang like an angel. At one point, I turned to Pete and said, "You know, if God wants to take me, this might be a good time." He just smiled back at me nodding his head.

Normally at an event like Gill's birthday party, I'd be close to the bar having several glasses of wine or whisky to soothe the nerves. I was on my way to the bar for my second glass of wine when I stopped in my tracks and said to myself, "Please, not tonight." I drank Diet Coke for the rest on the evening and because of that, I have a memory that will last a lifetime. Too many times, I let drink rob me of such precious moments.

I went back to Pete and Erin's house after the party and sat around their kitchen table as we replayed all that had unfolded in the previous few hours. Even by Pete and Erin's standards, which were high since they saw all the major country artists on a regular basis, we knew we had witnessed something special.

I got back to the hotel just before midnight but my brain was on fire. All in one magical day, I completed my first solo album with some of the world's finest musicians, and I had just come from the fiftieth birthday party of one of the top names in music. I didn't sleep too much that night.

The next morning, I met Pete and Erin at the Pancake Pantry Diner for a farewell breakfast before heading back to New Jersey. The diner was a legendary haunt for the Nashville music elite. I love diners so Pete promised to take me there once the album was complete. Over a delicious breakfast of some of the best pancakes I've ever had, we talked about what we accomplished in a few short days. I could tell Pete was proud of the CD. He had produced many instrumental CDs, but this was his first full-band and vocal CD. When Pete stepped away from the table, his wife Erin said, "Seamus, Pete gets very restless after recording an artist for more than a few days at a time, and more often than not, he's ready to move on to the next project. But he will miss working with you—he loves the way your album sounds." That was as high a compliment as I could get from the wife of someone whom I considered to be one of the world's finest guitar players, but also from someone highly respected in the music business in her own right.

Mission Accomplished

As I got back in my car to head north, I realized I had just had the most amazing week of my musical career. As I listened to the rough mix of the album, I knew the music had changed but the songs were still the same. Pete didn't try to make me into someone I was not, he just brought something out in me that I didn't know was there. I left Nashville a much better musician than I was seven short days earlier. I felt different. That flame that was ignited at the Bottom Line in 2002 was shining bright.

I took my time driving back to New Jersey. I stopped somewhere in West Virginia for the night. I needed time to absorb all that had transpired. I sat in a country bar staring into space wondering where my musical journey would take me next.

I arrived home late the next afternoon. I wanted to play the CD for Mary Pat immediately, but after a few songs, the little guys wanted me to play soccer. Young children have a way of bringing you back to reality in an instant. Later that evening, Mary Pat listened to the entire CD and liked what she heard. She remarked that the songs were still the same only better, picking up on my own feelings.

The CD was released on Memorial Day 2007. Blackthorn was doing a big outdoor show in Philly. They were gracious enough to let me add my CD to the band's merchandise table. It was an exhilarating feeling seeing people walking around with my CD. It really hit home when I was asked to sign the album during our break between sets. It felt very different than from when I signed the Blackthorn CDs every night. Four Cups of Coffee was my statement to the world of who I was at that moment in time. Blackthorn had a very busy schedule and I hoped to recoup some of the money for my investors within a month or so. Four days later, everything changed.

The Other Side of Town

"The Other Side of Town," by Seamus Kelleher"

There's a bell ringing out on the other side of town
It's calling my name but I ain't going down
I recognize the tune but I won't sing that song
I'm not ready for the Other Side of Town

A week after the album release was when I fell down the two flights of stairs at Kildare's Irish Pub. I was blessed to be with people who knew exactly what to do when they saw what happed. If someone other than the medics had tried to move me after the fall, it could have caused even more damage to my fractured skull. I was fortunate the fall happened next to a helipad that could accommodate a medevac chopper to transport me to one of the best trauma centers in America.

As I drifted in and out of consciousness on the medevac helicopter, I knew I had done something really stupid and I was on the verge of losing everything. I feared never seeing Mary Pat and my kids again. As crazy as it may sound, I was also sad I might never again perform the songs on my first solo album. My emotions were fueled by a combination of frustration, shame, depression and fear. I didn't fear death as much as letting my family down and not saying a proper goodbye to them. I also feared the loss of my mental capacity if I did survive. It was not the way I wanted my journey to end.

I had subdural hematomas or bleeding on both sides of the brain. In addition, I had some broken ribs and a bruised back. After three days in ICU, the doctors did a final CT scan before doing surgery to stop the bleeding. To their surprise, the bleeding had stopped in both locations. I was moved from the intensive care unit to the recovery ward and within a few days was discharged. I walked out of the hospital with the aid of a cane.

The first few weeks after the accident were excruciatingly difficult as the headaches were unbearable. I spent most of my time in bed. I got up once a day and went downstairs to eat with the kids so they would think things were somewhat normal. My oldest son, James, was nine years of age: old enough to know that things were not good. A few days after coming home from hospital, Mary Pat asked if I could play a short card game with him to reassure him I was alright. My speech was slurred, and I had trouble remembering the kids' names. I also had trouble putting full sentences together, but I told Mary Pat I'd give it a try. I'm not a card player, but I knew that James needed a sign. We just did one round of the game, which—on that rare occasion—I won. It was enough to reassure him I was on the road to recovery, and off he went to play with his toys.

Despite my card-game victory, there was a period during that first week at home when I was unsure I would make it. The headaches were relentless, especially when the pain meds wore off. I'm not a religious person, but I considered asking Mary Pat to call the local priest to give me the last rites. I believed I was heading for the "Other Side of Town."

A week after being discharged from the hospital, Mary Pat and I had a meeting with my neurosurgeon in Philadelphia. He didn't sugarcoat my situation. He took a plastic mold of the brain from his desk and explained in graphic detail that mine was badly bruised in the fall and there were parts of it permanently damaged. He looked at me and said, "Mr. Kelleher, you have been through a major trauma. You may be different moving forward. You can expect to have seizures and your cognitive abilities may be impaired. Only time will tell the long-term impact of the damage done to your brain." He didn't elaborate more than that, but he was basically preparing Mary Pat and me for the worst. It was a sobering moment for both of us. I wondered what Mary Pat was feeling. Was she angry and frustrated? I felt guilty for my stupidity but I also knew that to survive this, I had to focus on my recovery. It was indeed a traumatic event and I was damaged physically and mentally.

Recovery

After a few weeks at home, I was able to get out of bed and walk down the street with Mary Pat and the aid of a cane. The real turning point came several weeks after I got out of the hospital when my mother-in-law, Marge and her husband Joe, invited me, along with some of their friends, to accompany them on a week-long vacation at Goose Rocks Bay in Kennebunkport, Maine. I was reluctant to go as it involved a six-hour car ride and I didn't know how I could do that given the constant pain of the broken ribs and severe headaches. But I also knew I was slipping back into a deep depression and I needed a change of scenery, a sign of some kind of light, so I agreed to go. I made it through the long journey with the help of some painkillers and by positioning myself between multiple pillows Mary Pat strategically placed in the back of my in-laws' minivan.

When we got to Maine, I was still walking very gingerly, a few steps at a time, with the help of the walking stick. I was also on a high regimen of pain killers, making it necessary to nap every few hours. The hardest part of the week was the gap between when the meds wore off and when I could take my next dose.

Each day at Goose Rocks, I felt a little improvement. I'm sure part of the healing was due to being totally removed from the constant reminders of the accident and the quite solitude away from the day-to-day happenings of a busy household with four active children. The eight of us at the house in Goose Rocks Bay had wonderful conversations about life, politics and our trials and tribulations. They allowed me the time to form my sentences and thoughts, even though it took much longer than normal. When I struggled to find a missing word, they helped me without making me feel bad. It was an intellectual healing massage for my damaged brain. I was blessed to be in their loving and kind company. I could tell Joe and Marge were happy to see me re-engage. They were clearly concerned for my wellbeing, but they worried what life would be like for their daughter given the severity of my injuries. Would I be able to go back to work or play music? Would I be there for their four grandchildren?

I had my guitar with me in Maine and each evening I went out on the porch to play a few tunes. At first, I had difficulty forming the simplest of chords, but after a few days, I was able to play complete songs. While I struggled to remember things that had just happened the day before, I was able to recall the words of songs without any problem despite the fact I struggle with lyrics at the best of times. I went for a walk in the evenings and felt my body getting stronger. After a few days in Goose Rocks, I was walking over a mile at a time and the stabbing pain in my head subsided.

Mary Pat was shocked to see me walk in the door a week later without the use of the cane. She was delighted to see the life returning to my badly damaged body and, more importantly, my bruised brain. We both believed I'd most likely recover from my trauma, but we weren't sure what my new normal would be.

The brain is an amazing organ but even with all the advanced technology we have at our disposal today, there is much we don't know about how it functions. What we do know is that every head injury is different. In my case, the biggest challenge was my speech, especially when I was tired, which was most of the time. Four weeks after the accident, I still had a hard time pronouncing the most basic words and I found it difficult to form sentences, without taking extra time to make sure what I was saying wasn't gibberish.

In addition to her demanding schedule for Kelleher Creations, Mary Pat had to parent our four children. She had little time to internalize what had happened. What was going through her mind when she had to drive from Cranford, New Jersey to downtown Philly at 3 am after getting the call saying I had been medevacked to the trauma center? She never blamed me for my stupidity on that terrible night, even though she came very close to becoming a widow. Like me, she focused a hundred percent on my recovery.

The day after my accident, Mary Pat had to inform my work colleagues that I would not be coming into work that Monday. She looked through my phone contacts and called the only name she recognized: Michael Jalbert, the president of MRI. When I was in hospital, Jalbert came to visit me. A few weeks later, he sent an email asking me to come to his office for a visit. I wasn't exactly sure why, as I was in a fragile state and in no position to go back to work. It was also a two-hour journey from our home to the office. I was concerned about co-workers seeing me in my weakened state. Mary Pat came with me.

There were about forty people in the office when we got there in the early afternoon. I got a heartwarming welcome from everyone. Jalbert's assistant, Nadine, was delighted to see me and said the boss was waiting. After asking how I was doing, Jalbert told me to check in once a week by phone. What he was really doing was getting me off short-term disability and putting me back on the payroll, which guaranteed my full salary and insurance benefits would continue. He had no expectation of me doing any work until I was in a better place. I will never forget his kindness to me and my family during my time of need.

I did an open-air concert with Blackthorn in Philly six weeks after the fall. It was time to go back on stage, but I had no clue if I'd be able to

270

remember any of the songs. We were still a big deal in Philly, so there were a few thousand people at the show. The first thing I noticed upon my arrival at the venue was a temporary stage four feet off the ground with no railings. I was still walking very slowly and I felt unsteady on my feet after just a few minutes. It was a sweltering evening with temperature in the high 90s.

Before the show started, I called over our youngest roadie Colin and said, "Buddy, I need you to stand on the stage immediately to my right. If you see me going down, grab me and the guitar." Only a musician could say something as stupid as that. God forbid my prized Fender Stratocaster would take a tumble. In retrospect, I had no business being back on stage. It was too early, but somehow I made it through the two-hour show. I don't know if it was muscle memory or the mystery of the brain that I alluded to earlier, but everything came back to me. What helped me most that night was a sense of normalcy that came from playing with the band again. Blackthorn was truly a band of brothers and they were delighted to have me back on stage.

Around the same time, I went back to work at MRI. I immediately realized most of my written sentences were missing words and my spelling was terrible. I had a lady named Samantha working with me. She was a super-talented individual who helped me settle into MRI when I started. I told her that before anything went out from my desk, she had to proof and approve it. I asked her to keep our deal between the two of us. After a few months, I was able to take back control of the ship from Samantha.

Addiction

When I was in the hospital, the neurosurgeon strongly suggested I avoid alcohol moving forward. He cautioned that it could trigger seizures or worse. His message was loud and clear. I fully realized I dodged a bullet and swore I'd never take another drink. I was also aware I put my wife and children through enough. This was a golden opportunity to turn things around.

Six months after the accident, I figured it would be fine to have a glass of wine at dinner. Within a few weeks, one glass of wine turned into two and was soon joined by the odd Jameson whiskey. I come from a home where drinking was problematic, not just with my parents but back through generations of my family. The accident should have marked the end of my drinking forever, but alcoholism plays tricks on the mind. It's a deadly sickness.

From shortly after I started drinking in 1986 to the ride in the medevac chopper in 2007, there were numerous indications that I couldn't handle alcohol. People saw a successful executive, a talented guitar player with one of the most popular bands on the East Coast and a good dad to four children. They didn't see the horrible headaches that accompanied the weekend hangovers or the remorse I felt after making a fool of myself on stage. They were unaware of the squandered opportunities that came my way and the self-loathing that followed my bad behavior after a drinking session. They didn't see the pain I inflicted on Mary Pat and the disappointment in her face when I walked through the door drunk.

The Peoples' Band

By 2012, I knew it was time for me to move on from Blackthorn. We still performed in front of large crowds at festivals and clubs. It was a drinking culture and sometime that got in the way of potential success for the band. I wanted to leave Blackthorn when it was still somewhat fun. I completed a second solo album but didn't have an outlet to perform my music given the band's busy schedule. It was time to start a solo career, and I knew if I waited any longer, I'd be too old. After 17 years and over 1500 performances, I parted company with Blackthorn on the best of terms in 2012.

What made Blackthorn so special? We had a chemistry that kicked in every time we set foot on stage. Each band member gave their very best every night. We were more than a band; we were an institution in Philadelphia where multiple generations of families came to our shows. Our music was the soundtrack for family celebrations such as weddings, graduations and even the occasional wake. We were on TV and radio and were a mainstage attraction at some of the biggest festivals up and down the East Coast and the Midwest. Our manager, Jim McKee, was way ahead of his time constantly finding new opportunities for his bunch of misfits to extend their reach. We did three original albums. Sadly, an unwillingness to travel because of successful day jobs, and an abundance of well-paying local shows got in the way of us becoming a national act at the same level of Dropkick Murphy's and Flogging Molly. But we did break new ground and paved the way for many bands that came after us in the Pennsylvania, New Jersey and the New York metropolitan areas.

Depression

Less than a year after leaving Blackthorn, the parent company of MRI came under new management, and several senior executives were let go. I survived the first round of layoffs, but I knew it was only a matter of time before I was on the chopping block. I had an incredibly abusive boss at the parent company who took every opportunity to put me down. I had never experienced someone so obnoxious and rude in all my time in the corporate world. Day by day, I saw everything I worked so hard to build slip away. It was hard to fathom just six months earlier I was the recipient of the President's Leadership Award for helping the company navigate the financial crisis and recession of 2008.

I couldn't or at least thought I couldn't resign from MRI as I had four young children to take care of. I woke up every morning feeling like my chest was about to explode. On Fridays leaving work, I felt a weight lift off my shoulders but that feeling of dread came back late on Saturday and all-day Sunday. I was rapidly losing weight as I had no appetite for food and just picked at meals.

My sister Toni and her husband Martan were visiting from Ireland around the time I was feeling unwell. She could see I was in distress. I asked her, "When do you know it's time to get help?" She said, "If you are asking the question Seamus, then it's time."

A week before asking Toni when I needed help, I met a dear friend Jo for lunch and as soon as he saw me he said, "Seamus, what's wrong, brother? You're not yourself." He recognized I was in a bad way and told me in no uncertain terms I had to get the hell away from the job before it killed me.

Many times, it's our friends and family who recognize our struggles and pain before we do. Eventually I did go to my doctor who immediately put me on anxiety medication and suggested I see a psychiatrist. He also recommended I go on sick leave which I did two days later—but it was too late.

By Saturday, I experienced the worst depression and anxiety since my days In St. Patrick's hospital in Ireland in 1974. I was scheduled to perform at a party for some good friends that afternoon. On the way to the party, about ten miles from home, I pulled the car over. I had a full-blown panic attack. My heart was racing and I was sweating. I felt like I was trying to escape a burning building while being consumed by flames. I was certain my life was about to end.

I took some anxiety medication and after twenty minutes walking aimlessly around the car, I managed to get back on the road and made my way to the party. I had no idea if I could perform and was on the verge of bawling. I did my best to conceal the situation from my friends. I decided that if things didn't improve, I'd make an early exit from the party saying I had stomach problems. Somehow, I got through the afternoon. It helped that my friends were great singers, and they sang their hearts out with me during the show. Music is such a powerful healing force in my life. Just when things seem hopeless, it shows up and pulls me out of the darkness if only for a short time. That day, the music and my wonderful friends bought me some time.

When I got home, I didn't have to say a word to Mary Pat. She saw the frightened desperate look on my face. The anxiety that was building over several weeks was now accompanied by a deep depression. As always, Mary Pat listened and did her best to console me, but I was drowning in tears of sadness.

The next morning, things were worse. It's hard to explain what it feels like to be at such a low point in your life. Dr. Quinnett, a psychologist who has been an advocate for suicide prevention in the U.S. most of his life, said, "Suicide is what happens when pain exceeds hope." That Sunday morning, I lost all hope and the pain was unbearable. I didn't want to be in pain anymore and I didn't want to be a burden to Mary Pat and my lovely children. To be clear, I didn't take any steps to end my life. Knowing what I know now about suicide, I would consider what was going through my head as suicide ideation where you imagine not being here anymore, but you don't have a plan or even a desire to end your life by suicide. You are just trying to escape that burning building.

Mary Pat, in the most pragmatic way, said it was time to go to the emergency room at Doylestown Hospital, a few miles from our house. Like my Dad all those years ago in Ireland and my aunt Nora in Brooklyn, Mary Pat was smart enough to know I was in crisis and that immediate action was needed. Her inner strength that day, despite the worry and fear she was experiencing, heled me find the light.

The staff at the hospital emergency room recognized I was in a bad way and set about getting me admitted to a mental health facility in the area. After several hours, they found a room for me at Horsham Clinic, about ten miles from our home. But they couldn't admit me until much later that evening. Once I knew I had somewhere to go for help, I settled down a little and the sense of panic eased.

After we came back home from the hospital, we sat the kids down and Mary Pat told them I was sick and was going away for a while to get better. As I looked at their beautiful innocent faces, I was distraught that I was causing them worry and stress at such tender ages. They ranged in age from eight' to 14 years. There was no outburst of tears, but it was clear

276

they were concerned. Before setting off for the hospital, I hugged James, Rory, Nora and Aidan. I didn't want to let go. Would I be there to see James graduate high school, or to watch Aidan play baseball? Would I see Nora dress up for her prom? Would I hear Rory play music again in school? I didn't have answers to those questions.

At 6 pm, we set off for Horsham Clinic. The lush green lawns, beautiful trees and spectacular flower beds on each side of the driveway of the clinic were in stark contrast to the grayness I was feeling inside. It was a déjà vu moment as it was almost forty years since I drove up the driveway to St. Pat's hospital in Dublin.

Horsham Clinic was quiet as it was a Sunday evening, but the admissions process took a long time. It hit me hard what was happening when the medical staff took all sharp objects away from me including the belt for my pants and my shoelaces. Given my condition, they were worried I would try and harm myself. I was considered suicidal.

My memories of those first few days in the hospital are filled with darkness. I was in a ward with some folks who were a lot worse off than me. I was scared and my mind was racing. I woke up several times during the night to the sound of fighting and yelling and eventually police were called to the unit to restore order. After a few days, I was moved to a different unit which consisted of folks struggling with depression, anxiety, cutting, addiction and other mental health issues.

The staff at Horsham were fantastic. I was blessed to have an Irish lady, Jacinta Harman, taking care of me. She was also from Galway and was as tough as they come. If I didn't get out of bed at 6:30 am after the first wake-up call, I could her thick Irish brogue outside my room saying, "Kelleher, you're not in Galway now, it's time to get out of bed." She was my guardian angel and kept a close eye on me throughout my stay at the clinic.

Our days at Horsham were structured with group sessions where everyone on the ward shared their struggles. It was eye-opening to hear what others were dealing with. In many cases, their stories were harrowing. They talked openly about their daily struggles and in some cases how their families were being torn apart by their illness.

We supported each other when we could, and we often cried when it just got too hard to handle the pain. Each of us met regularly with our therapist and psychiatrist. There were many activities to occupy our minds, but like St. Pat's, the best part of the day was when we went to the nurse's station to receive the meds. You just hoped they would kick in so you could sleep that night—so you could escape the invisible pain.

After several days at Horsham, I felt much better. The depression was lifting, and the anxiety was almost gone. I had a meeting with the psychiatrist, Jacinta and Mary Pat and expected to be released from Horsham that afternoon. It was like a parole hearing. I did everything to convince them that I was fully back to "normal." I was joking around and smiling, but the smile was quickly wiped off my face when the psychiatrist stopped me in my tracks saying, "Seamus, you are very sick, and have a long way to go before it's safe for you to go home." To my surprise, Mary Pat and Jacinta nodded in total agreement. I was devastated. The psychiatrist explained that I had experienced a trauma and I needed time for healing to take place. She was also concerned I might harm myself. I wasn't happy. As Mary Pat said goodbye, putting on her bravest face and holding back the tears, she gave me an envelope with handwritten letters from each of our children. I read those beautiful pages from my children over and over. They told me about their music, school, the sports they played and how much they missed me. Those letters were better than and medicine and gave me reason to fight even harder so I could recover. I could empathize with what Mam went through when she got very sick after I was born. She had to fight hard to survive but now it was my time.

Two weeks before I was admitted to Horsham, Mary Pat started a full-time position with a large telecommunications company. She still managed to visit me every day at Horsham after work. In addition to a new job and worrying about me, she took care of the children, keeping life as normal as possible for them.

Mary Pat brought the kids to visit me after a week in hospital. We talked for a while and they could see I was doing better. It was hard on Mary Pat. Just a few years earlier, she had to deal with me in the intensive care unit of the University of Pennsylvania Trauma Unit not knowing if I was going to make it. This time, she wondered if I would find my way back from the darkness.

I wasn't allowed to have my guitar at the clinic as the strings could be used in a suicide attempt. But there was a room at Horsham with an upright piano. After much persuasion, Jacinta allowed me to play for a while. I think it was when Mary Pat heard I was playing piano that she knew I was on the mend.

During my stay at Horsham, Mary Pat asked our oldest son James if he had noticed I wasn't well prior to going into hospital. Without a moment's hesitation, he said, "Mom, when you don't hear dad playing guitar on the couch in the evening, you know it's not normal." We all have our diagnostic tools but sometimes the little things are the telltale signs something is not right. James nailed it and, to this day, my enthusiasm or lack of it for the guitar is probably the best barometer of my mental state. It's more accurate than any medical test.

Fellow Travelers

This may sound strange, but some amazing things happen when you are in a mental health facility over time. You form bonds with people who are struggling with their own demons even though their battles are very different from yours. You share each other's wins and losses, big or small; you grieve together, cry together, and become cheerleaders for each other. That was the case in both Horsham and at St. Pat's in Dublin forty years earlier. I was one of many in the fight of our lives.

After ten days at Horsham, I was discharged. But that was only the beginning of my recovery. There was a long road ahead. The following Monday, I began a three-week rigorous outpatient program at the clinic. It was five days a week from 9 am to 4 pm. I was one of 25 patients, some of whom had been inpatients for a week or more at Horsham, but there were others who had not been hospitalized or who had come from other mental health facilities.

The majority of sessions were geared towards providing coping mechanisms to help us assimilate back into the "real world." In addition to group meetings, we each had private consultations with a psychiatrist, which I found interesting and beneficial.

The first thing we did each morning was answer a questionnaire on how we were feeling on a scale of 1 to 10 and if we had any thoughts of harming ourselves. A few days after we started the program, a young man sitting next to me seemed very upset when he arrived at the facility. He got agitated when it came time for him to speak. He said in a quivering voice, "I drove here today and hit 100 MPH and went through several red lights and stop signs. I just want it to be over." For this young man, once again, pain exceeded hope. He had just described a suicide attempt in horrifying detail. As soon as he finished speaking, an assistant came over and brought him out of the classroom so he could speak to a therapist. I don't remember him coming back.

A New Chapter

"It can take a year and often longer to recover from a traumatic event and especially a trauma that involves your mental health." Those were the words I heard from a counselor during a group therapy session a month after I finished my treatment at Hosham. It's probably the wisest comment I've ever heard uttered by a mental health professional. During the session, I was full of pep telling the therapist I wanted to get back to work and also to my music. She told me to put the brakes on and give myself time to heal.

I was still on sick leave from MRI. After chatting with Mary Pat, we decided it would be a good idea for me to go back to Ireland for a few weeks to recuperate and spend time with my sisters and their families. I was there a few days and starting to feel much better when I got a call from my boss at MRI telling me my position was being eliminated. In some ways, I felt an enormous sense of relief that I wouldn't have to go back to work under such stressful circumstances. But I was also angry about being let go while still on sick leave. It was wrong on so many levels. I had given a lot to the company during my six-year tenure.

In my leadership role at MRI, I travelled all over the U.S., Europe and Asia visiting various offices and making some lifelong friends along the way. I managed a wonderful team of young people who always found a way to make things happen. After Michael Jalbert left MRI, I worked directly for Tony McKinnon, the next president of the company and a natural leader. He brought out the best in me and always positioned me for success. We became dear friends. It was after he retired that things went downhill for me at MRI. It was by far the best day job I ever had. It was hard not having an opportunity to say a proper goodbye to my friends and colleagues. It was a sad and abrupt end to a wonderful chapter in my life.

Finding my Voice

After recovering from my illness, I started back doing some local shows. I was still trying to figure out who I was as a solo musician. My stage craft needed a lot of work plus the money for each show was less than half of what I made with Blackthorn. When Blackthorn fans came to see me, many were a little disappointed as my gigs paled in comparison to the highly produced Blackthorn shows. Many of them felt sorry for me. In particular, I remember a family of die-hard Blackthorn fans coming to see me. They were very nice but I could tell they didn't enjoy what I was doing. Of course, they didn't say anything, but the look on their faces and their body language spoke volumes. They wondered why I left one of the most successful bands in the country with roadies and managers, playing to thousands of people in large venues, to play in small bars in the Doylestown area with just an acoustic guitar in hand.

I got a part-time consulting job at Philadelphia Gas Works. I was doing an analysis of the communications at the company. The job was a great boost to my confidence, which was shattered after being fired from MRI. The job allowed me to put a routine in my day and that helped my mental state enormously. As I was finishing up the consulting job, I got a call from Lincoln Financial, a big insurance company, asking me to come in for an interview as speech writer for the president.

I walked into Lincoln Financial's corporate headquarters excited but wondering if I still had what it took to survive and thrive in such a fast-paced environment. The president Will Fuller was full of life and passionate about his work and his people. He was from down South and had that wonderful southern drawl and the charm to go with it. We talked for over an hour sharing our thoughts on leadership and a variety of other topics. When I left his office, I knew I had accomplished a lot by being able to engage with the president of a major financial institution.

A day later, human resources at Lincoln called to extend an offer to me. I was stunned and relieved that once again I would have a steady income with great benefits.

Aged Out

The work at Lincoln was very different from what I had done before. I had to learn an entirely new industry at age 58 and it was daunting. My direct boss, who was in charge of communications, was very fair but the pressure on us both to deliver the goods was stressful. I was in charge of writing all the speeches for the president. So here I was, writing remarks on a topic I was clueless about. Maybe if I were younger, or if my mental state was more stable, I would have been up to the task, but I never felt comfortable in the job even though it lasted two years.

It was clear to me—and to my boss—that I was way out of my league at Lincoln Financial. In addition, I had extreme pain in both shoulders, which the doctor diagnosed as tendinitis with some spurs. I could barely lift my hands to get something from a high shelf in our kitchen and found it difficult to get dressed in the morning. It was also interfering with my music engagements as I struggled to lift the equipment in and out of venues. I ended up having shoulder surgery, which forced me to take time off from Lincoln.

When I went back to work after the surgery, I found myself drinking more, sometimes stopping for a few drinks on my home from work. I also increased my alcohol intake in the evenings. I had that same dread of going to work on a Monday morning that I experienced in my final days at MRI. I was seeing the early signs of depression and anxiety come back with a vengeance. Things reached a peak while on the way to work one morning, I fell asleep on a crowed highway. I was on antidepressants and I had taken anxiety meds before leaving home. I was awoken by the noise from the rumble strips on the side of the road and somehow managed to maintain control of my car. Once again, it felt like the end of the road.

Sobriety

On Halloween in 2014, Mary Pat took our youngest out for trick or treat. The others, too old for the annual ritual, were at home celebrating Rory's birthday with his friends. Later in the evening, Mary Pat set up an elaborate candy scavenger hunt for the kids in our back yard. After playing for hours, they came inside. They all played musical instruments, some in the school band. For over an hour they had a jam session like no other with all kinds of hoots and hollers. There was piano, guitar, sax, trumpet, trombone and cajon. Sadly, it's all a blurry memory as I had way too much to drink.

Before Mary Pat came home from work, I had a few whiskies as I knew two glasses of wine in the evening wasn't going to get me where I wanted to be. I also went next door to the neighbor's house for some more wine while Mary Pat had Aidan out trick-or-treating in the neighborhood. When I returned home and throughout the evening, Mary Pat asked if I was okay. I was repeating myself and getting emotional. At times I was totally incoherent.

When the kids were to be picked up by their parents, Mary Pat suggested several times that I should head up to bed. She wasn't angry with me as I wasn't falling-down drunk, but she thought it would be better if the parents didn't see me inebriated. Eventually I went to bed and within moments was in a deep alcohol-induced sleep.

I woke early the next morning. I wasn't hung over but I was feeling incredibly sad. I asked myself what was I doing to my kids and Mary Pat? Dark memories of my own childhood when I constantly worried about drinking on the home front flashed vividly through my mind like it was yesterday. I burst into tears and said, "It's now or never Seamus."

I picked up the phone and called my good friend Mike Brill—a fellow musician who was sober then for over ten years. I said, "Mike, I have a problem with the drink." Those are the most important and honest words that ever came out of my mouth. For the first time in over thirty years of drinking, I admitted I was an alcoholic and I was ready to stop. My friend Ella was right when she told me I was an alcoholic many years earlier—I just wasn't ready to listen and admit it.

Within hours of our phone call, Mike came to the house. In addition to being a recovering alcoholic, he is a substance abuse counselor. He listened as I shared how bad the drinking had become and how I feared I would lose everything if I didn't make a change. There was no judgment in his voice when he said, "Okay buddy, let's move forward and find the "Light."

During a meeting for alcoholics at a local church the following day, I uttered the words, "My name is Seamus, I'm an alcoholic, I've been sober for 36 hours." As soon as the words escaped my lips, I could hear them reverberate as if I were in an echo chamber. The genie was out of the bottle. At the time of writing, I've been sober almost seven years.

I'm sure Mary Pat wondered how long my sobriety would last. After all, I had tried to stop drinking before and managed to do so for months at a time. This time around, I didn't talk about it to Mary Pat. I knew it was time to walk the talk. Too many promises had been broken in the past, starting with our wedding day when I got drunk halfway through the reception. So many fun evenings when we gathered together with friends and family ended with me being drunk. More often than not, I had little recollection of what had happened when I woke up the next morning. There were many birthdays and celebrations where I was not present.

The trust between Mary Pat and myself was gone and had to be earned back. I couldn't undo the hurt I had caused with my years of alcohol abuse, but I had an opportunity to salvage our marriage and rebuild a life without alcohol. I didn't apologize to Mary Pat then for what I put her through and in retrospect I should have. But I had promised to curb my drinking so many times before and it never happened. This time around, I felt my actions were more import than words.

When did I know I was an alcoholic? If I'm being totally honest, I would say within a year of taking my first drink in 1986. I knew early on I could not control my drinking, but it took so long to admit it because I knew by doing so, I'd have to quit. I didn't want to lose my best friend, even though my friend was slowly killing me and ruining every aspect of my life.

I bet if you ask most people who knew me during my drinking years if they thought I had a problem with drink, they would say no. What they might say is, "Seamus used to have a good time when he was drinking but I never saw him out of control." What my friends didn't see was the damage the drink was doing.

I know I can never make up to Mary Pat for what I put her through. There were many nights when she stayed up late worrying where I was or what shape I'd come home in. I'm sure she wondered if our children would get to know their Dad as adults. She deserved better.

Goodbye to Corporate Life

About a year into my sobriety, Mary Pat saw a job opening at Drexel University for a speech writer for the president. With my academic background, it seemed like a much better fit for me than Lincoln Financial. I did a few interviews and was offered the job of Executive Director of Executive and Strategic Communications—by far the best and most ridiculous job title I've ever held.

As I said goodbye to my co-workers at Lincoln, I wondered if Drexel would be different or if I had aged out of the corporate world. A few weeks into the job, I had my answer. Once again, I was in way over my head. I was in no way qualified to do what was expected of me. Since Drexel was expanding its footprint in the Philadelphia area, there was a lot of work to be done with the city administration and at the state level in Harrisburg. It was totally outside of my area of expertise. Maybe if I were younger, I would have been up to the challenge. I was totally deflated, and it began to dawn on me I couldn't do it anymore.

I did my best to rise to the challenges of the job but each day things got progressively worse. I knew my superiors were not happy with my job performance. I felt ashamed to tell Mary Pat what was going on.

I arrived home from work one evening and went straight up to the bedroom without saying anything to her or the kids. I was angry at myself for ending up again in a situation where I felt I failed at my job. What the hell was wrong with me? When Mary Pat came upstairs to the bedroom, I was sitting on the bed sobbing. She just held me as the anguish gradually subsided. She could see I was hurting deep inside.

Mary Pat dropped me at the train station the next morning. Just before I got out of the car, she said with a concerned look on her face, "Are you okay?" to which I answered, "I'm a few days away from going back to Horsham." She looked me straight in the eye and said, "You need to resign today." We both knew it was time.

Later that morning, I asked for a meeting with my boss. I told her I was aware the job was not a good fit and they were not getting what Drexel expected and needed from me. We both agreed that the position as it had evolved was different from what I had interviewed for. We had a wonderful conversation and figured out a way forward.

I emerged from the meeting with a commitment that I would resign, but I would stay on for several weeks and train someone in the art of speechwriting. As part of the understanding, I was given a generous severance package. Also, the university paid for a career consultant to help me find my way forward.

As I walked out of Drexel's beautiful and ornate Main building, I felt a calm come over me like nothing I've ever experienced in my entire life. By the time I got to the train for my hour-and a-half commute home, the stress and anxiety that was taking such a toll began to lift like a morning fog

I parted company with Drexel on the best of terms. I received a lovely personal note from John Fry, the president of the university, thanking me for the support I provided him during my short tenure.

A Way Forward

A few weeks later I met with Sue, my career counselor. After a few sessions, we agreed that my time as an executive in the corporate world was done. I had a 17-year career with several great companies, working and learning from some incredible people along the way. I went from being a low-level consultant at EDS in 1995 to being Vice President of Marketing and Communications at MRI in 2008. But my final corporate years made it clear that it was time to find a different path.

I told Sue I wanted to focus on my music and maybe do some marketing consulting work. She agreed and we set about putting a plan in place to achieve my goals. I knew there was a lot of work ahead but I felt an incredible sense of relief and optimism.

Over the course of the next several months, I increased the number of music gigs. I invested in a better sound system and additional equipment to make my show more fun and suitable for larger venues. I also incorporated the electric guitar into my shows and that was an instant game changer. I found my niche.

In 2016, I started working part time at the Foundry marketing agency in Doylestown. They gave me a space to work in their office, and that helped me get up and moving and out of the house each morning. It was great being surrounded by creative folks I could bounce ideas off.

Over the course of the last four years, I've gone from doing 60 shows a year to 200 in 2019. I travel across the country from Colorado, Kansas and Indiana to New York, New Jersey, Maryland and Florida. In addition to performing, I do my motivational talk Shine the Light where I share my experiences of dealing with depression, anxiety and alcohol addiction.

Mental Wellness

While the vast majority of days are good for me, I have the occasional times when I get down. I have an agreement with my psychiatrist, whom I see once a year, that if I experience more than three or four bad days in a row, he gets a call from me so we can take immediate action. I also struggle with type 2 diabetes. I have it under control but I have my blood checked a few times a year and if my a1c (blood sugar level) starts climbing, I see my doctor right away. Why wouldn't I take the same approach with my mental health? That may sound incredibly pragmatic but that's how we need to think in terms of our mental wellness if we are to address the scourge of suicide in this country—over 47,500 deaths in 2019.

We all can play a role in helping those who struggle. Some of the warning signs to watch for:

- Talking of suicide or wanting to die
- Loss of hope and no reason to live
- No joy in life
- Sleeping too much or too little
- Increased agitation and irritability
- Increased use of drugs and alcohol
- A feeling of being a burden to others
- Extreme mood changes and deep sadness
- Preoccupation with death
- Acting anxious, agitated or reckless

When I come across someone who exhibits signs of distress, I employ the widely used QPR (Question-Persuade-Refer) suicide prevention protocol. It was developed by Dr. Paul Quinnett in the 1990s to help those who were suicidal, but it's a great way of helping anyone who is experiencing a crisis in their life even if they are not suicidal. I have used the protocol many times to help people battling addiction.

If you do see someone who is struggling with their mental wellness or addiction and fear for their safety, don't be afraid to ask the difficult *Question*: "Are you considering harming yourself?" Offer words of encouragement and try to *Persuade* them to get help. Better still, take them or *Refer* them to a crisis center, a doctor's office or a hospital emergency room where they can get the professional help they desperately need. Don't try to be their therapist. Your job is to persuade them to get the help they need.

Many times, folks fear losing a friendship by asking tough questions when a friend is in crisis. I'd rather lose a friendship any day than a friend. But the reality is, most people in crisis will have a positive reaction when you reach out to them and offer support. You might just save a life by asking that simple question: "Are you okay?" You can find out more about the QPR suicide prevention protocol at qprinstitute.com.

The National Suicide Prevention Lifeline telephone number should be in all our phones. They are trained to deal with people who are in crisis and can direct them to the help they desperately need. As of the time of writing, that number is 1-800-273-8255 (Note that the number is scheduled to be changed to 988 in 2022). There is also a Crisis Text line where 24/7 support is available. That number is 741741.

The Big Wheel of Life

The year 2020 was scheduled to be the best of my musical career. I had over two hundred shows booked, including a sold-out bus tour of Ireland in June 2020. But everything came to crashing halt on March 15 when Pennsylvania along with much of America and the rest of the world went into lockdown because of the Corona virus.

Within days, two of my children came home from college and continued their studies online. My youngest, Aidan, in the spring term of his junior year, also started his classes online. Because of her position in the telecom business, Mary Pat was deemed an essential worker so she was busier than ever.

I looked at my music calendar and realized all those dates I had worked so hard to book were gone. I felt like everything I built over several years vanished in the blink of an eye. Like everyone, I was fearful about the future. Nobody knew for sure how bad the pandemic was or how long it would last. The 24-hour news cycle with its constant doom and gloom made it hard to get up in the morning. It was compounded by a presidential election that grew more contentious by the day, adding to our nation's heightened anxiety.

Two weeks into the lockdown, I got a call from Dr. Lori Wick, the Assistant Dean for Student Affairs at Texas A&M College of Medicine, where I had given my "Shine the Light" talk in 2018. She asked if I would talk to the staff and faculty as they struggled to deal with their new reality as a result of the pandemic. I had two days to prepare. I titled my talk "Mental Wellness in Times of Crisis." I did the presentation over the Zoom platform, which I had never used before. I opened up the talk by singing "The Gambler," a song from Kenny Rogers, the much-loved Texas native who passed a few days earlier.

The theme of my talk was to let people know we would get through this crisis but there were things we needed to focus on to come out on the other side. I gave examples of how I had managed through some of my darkest days dealing with depression, anxiety and addiction by getting help when I needed it. I stressed the importance of watching for the warning signs that you might be in trouble.

The faculty and staff liked the presentation. Later in the day, I got another call from Dr. Wick asking if I would consider putting together a two-week class for their medical students focused on the same topic. I said yes and had two days to develop a syllabus and to master the dreaded Zoom technology.

I was delighted to be back teaching. My last class at New York University was in 2007. This was not the way I expected to get back into teaching, but it was an incredible opportunity to do something I love and help people in the process. As of today, I've completed twelve classes at Texas A&M College of Medicine. In addition to the Mental Wellness class, I also teach courses on suicide prevention. Two months into my teaching assignment, I was appointed to the Texas A&M College of Medicine part-time faculty as an adjunct assistant professor. My Mental Wellness course is now an elective for all medical students and the plan is for it to continue long after the virus has passed. Being back teaching has given me a great sense of purpose. It was meant to be. I'm bringing together the skills I've honed throughout my life and helping those who struggle in the process.

During the pandemic, I also did several presentations in the corporate world where I talked about the importance of mental wellness. I incorporate musical performances into each talk. While the topic of mental wellness in heavy, the music relaxes the audience and allows the message to get across in a non-threatening manner. These talks have led to many opportunities in the post pandemic world.

Like most people, I had some very dark days in 2020. But having all four children home was a gift in the midst of the darkness. We helped each other get through the hard days and found joy in our great extended dinner conversations and our post-dinner board games which often lasted for hours.

The Reset

The lockdown during Covid was an opportunity to reflect on my life and do a reset. I realized I was doing way too many shows leaving little time for Mary Pat and the kids. Also, I didn't have time to feed my creative side. Over the past twelve months, I've started writing music again for the first time in years. Moving forward, I plan on doing more teaching and motivational talks and I've cut down on live performances. I might even do another book.

Despite my struggles with mental health and addiction, I've lived a life full of adventure with all the ups and downs that come along with that. I performed a sold-out concert at Carnegie Hall with the Sean Fleming Band. I've met Bono and the Edge and I've shared the stage with the Saw Doctors, the Pogues and Thin Lizzy.

I've worked at jobs that stretched me to my limit—sometimes it worked and sometimes I failed miserably. I go on stage every night not knowing how crowds will react to my music, but there are many nights I get a standing ovation with people one-third my age going crazy. I still get that same exhilarating feeling when I perform I got during that Young You talent competition at the Claddagh Hall in Galway in 1970.

Most of all, I've been blessed to re-establish my relationship with my beautiful and talented wife, Mary Pat, and our four funny, smart and incredibly kind children. I learn from them each day although I've been cancelled a few times!

When I look in the mirror today, I see a senior citizen whose hair has mostly turned gray. But I also see someone who is at peace—someone who is fully embracing life—someone with a purpose who wants to Shine the Light for those who are trying to find their way out of the darkness. I pray there will be many more stops on my journey but I'm thankful for all the good Lord has provided me.

Now it's time to go practice my guitar playing. I have a big show tomorrow. I want to give it my best.

The End

Acknowledgements

To my wife, Mary Pat—thank you for hanging in there, even during the darkest of times when I didn't merit the support and love you gave me. Your encouragement, your probing questions and your editing skills have helped get my story down on paper.

To my children—James, Rory, Nora and Aidan—I don't know if you will every fully know how much I love you. You are the shining lights that kept me going. I'm so proud of who you've become.

To Mike Farragher, author, motivational speaker, playwright, screenwriter and my writing mentor—thank you for showing me how to write a book. I'm forever grateful for your guidance and encouragement.

To Gay Adelman who allowed me to find my voice and provided invaluable guidance on how to bring my stories to life. I still hear you saying, "Seamus, take me there, tell me how it felt. Paint the picture."

To Niall O'Dowd who believed in me from my early days in New York. You provided me with many opportunities throughout my career. I went dark for many years but when I emerged from behind the clouds, you picked up where we left off and allowed me to tell my story in your wonderful publications. I'm honored to call you a friend.

To Cahal Dunne, you have been such an inspiration to me on so many levels. I'm a better musician and entertainer because of you. I can't count how many texts I got from you in the past twelve months saying,

"How is the book coming along, Seamus?" It was your gentle Cork way of saying, "Get the darn thing finished."

To Larry Kirwan, author, playwright, radio host and master entertainer who has always been there to support me and encourage me to take risks in order to accomplish what seemed impossible.

To Shannon Diffner who took my manuscript and transformed it into something I could only have dreamed of. You have a special gift. Thanks for letting me be the beneficiary of your many talents.

To Govan Martin, the chair and executive director of the Suicide Prevention Alliance, who fights tirelessly to help those who are suicidal and those impacted by suicide—I treasure our friendship and I'm a better teacher because of you.

To Andy McEntee, Chris Ebneth, Sean Fleming, Chris Bishop, Jacinta Harman, Andrejs E. Avots-Avontis, Gerry Hanberry, David Cazabon, PJ Duggan, Marco Magliocco, Damien Hanley, Eileen Rogers Brown, and my wonderful in-laws Joe and Marge Shields and countless others—thanks for taking the time to review or provide input to the manuscript and for all the suggestions that have helped make the book what it is.

To Erin Morris Huttlinger: I miss your husband Pete more than you know, but I could feel his presence when I was writing this book. I know he would be proud of me. Working with you, helped propel me along when things got tough over the past few years.

To Karen Bloomfield, whose eagle-eyed editing and proofing skills make it possible to read this book without going blind: I value your talent and our friendship.

To Mike Brill: thanks for helping me see the Light of sobriety. I am forever grateful to you, my friend.

Thanks to Paul Prizer for the wonderful cover. Also, a special thank you to my friends at Minuteman Press in Doylestown for all your support.

To Dr. Lori Wick at Texas A&M College of Medicine. You reminded me time after time of the importance of getting this book done even when I wanted to walk away from it. I gained much insight into the medical profession and its practitioners during our weekly conversations.

To my sisters Geraldine, Carol, Maura and Toni and your beautiful families: I can't imagine what my life would be like without you. Mam and Dad gave us an incredible gift, a closeness that has endured for almost seven decades. I treasure what we have and I never take it for granted.

To Mam and Dad: you both left this world way too early. What I would give for you to meet Mary Pat and our children. I know they would see what my sisters and I saw: two of the kindest people who have ever walked the earth. When the days are hard and the nights are dark, I think of you and draw from that bottomless well of love and kindness you provided my sisters and I growing up in Galway.

Reviews

In Shine the Light, Seamus Kelleher shares with readers his very personal story of excelling as a gifted guitarist and performer, all the while battling depression, anxiety and alcohol addiction. He conveys his message openly and honestly, sharing his life experiences in a way that the reader can identify with, helping to normalize issues related to mental health. His story gives the reader a unique insight into depression, anxiety and addiction. It is also inspirational, providing hope for those battling the same demons.

Lori Wick, MD, Assistant Dean at Texas A&M College of Medicine

Shine The Light is the perfect metaphor for the amazing life of Celtic rocker and mental well-being adjunct professor Seamus Kelleher. From his early trauma of sadistic priests and teachers in the Ireland of the 1960s and '70s almost destroying his self-esteem, to just barely surviving alcoholism, deep depression and brain surgery, he should be dead. But he survived it all due to his soul-saving guitar, his brutal honesty and tenacity, the love and patience of his wife, children, parents, sisters and relatives, and his amazingly kind friends and colleagues. Shine The Light is a must-read for anyone who is losing hope.

Cahal Dunne, Musician and Author

Seamus has written a fine book about the art of survival. It's not pretty, it's often brutally honest, but it tells the story of a very talented working musician who never complained about the hand that was dealt him in an unforgiving Ireland. Seamus has survived his demons but they're never far from hand. He's come a long way, but I can't help thinking of that fresh-faced Galway boy I first met up around Kingsbridge Road in the Bronx who went on to become a hero. Read this book, it will do you a world of good, and pass it on to someone else when you're finished. It's a tonic for the soul.

Larry Kirwan, Founding member of Black 47, Radio Host, Composer, Playwright and Author

A gifted and talented musician, Seamus Kelleher shares his journey as a musician and the associated highs and lows of a career as a performer. His struggles with anxiety, depression and addiction are an added burden and reflect the complications in both his personal and professional life. His story is one of hope and resilience and sends the message that the stigma of mental health shouldn't be a hurdle to asking for and receiving help.

Andrejs E. Avots-Avotins, MD, PhD;

Vice President Medical Affairs Baylor Scott & White Health

Life was grim for this sensitive youth as he moved through his early teenage years in a small seaside town in the far West of Ireland in the early 1970s. Traumatised by the terrifying brutalities he encountered daily in his school and burdened by feelings of inadequacy, young Seamus Kelleher was struggling to get through as best he could from day to day until that magical afternoon when he picked up a guitar for the very first time and his life changed forever. This book tells the fascinating story of that extraordinary life, a life lived by the maxim that one should "follow one's dreams wherever they lead." But part of this great dream also involves the darkest of nightmares including serious depression, fragility, confinements and the horrors of alcoholism. With an honesty and openness that is extraordinary and compelling, Seamus outlines his difficult struggle to overcome these demons. This is a terrific and inspiring story operating on many levels and will enthral the reader from the opening page to the final paragraph.

Gerry Hanberry, Educator, Author and Poet

Amy Winehouse once said, "every bad situation is a blues song waiting to happen," and you can hear that truth in every fiery blue guitar lick that howls from Seamus Kelleher's fret board. His life was not an easy one and like many a rock star before him, it must be said that he sometimes made his life way harder than it had to be. He has scaled dizzying heights and pillaged the continents on never ending tours, living a life few could scarcely dream about it and has been seared by the spotlight. He has taken the time to look back and chronicled this colorful journey in a book that is at times raw, witty, brave, and mischievous. His unflinching portrayal of the hard times paves the way for others to tell his truth, which makes him a hero of not just the guitar.

Mike Farragher, Author, Columnist, TV Producer and Motivational Speaker

About the Author

Master storyteller and guitarist Seamus Kelleher has been performing in venues across the US and Europe for close to fifty years. Through his career, he has battled depression, anxiety and an addiction to alcohol. Seamus is committed to helping those who struggle and removing the stigma of mental illness and addiction. He is an Adjunct Assistant Professor at Texas A&M College of Medicine where he teaches courses on Mental Wellness and Suicide Prevention. He continues to entertain audiences with his unforgettable Celtic rock and blues show. In addition, Seamus engages audiences across America with his motivational talk, "Shine the Light."

Made in United States
Orlando, FL
18 November 2021